Practical Ethics for General Practice

Practical Ethics for General Practice

SECOND EDITION

Wendy A Rogers
Department of Medical Education, Flinders University

and

Annette J Braunack-Mayer
Discipline of Public Health, University of Adelaide

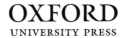

OXFORD
UNIVERSITY PRESS

OXFORD

UNIVERSITY PRESS

Great Clarendon Street, Oxford OX2 6DP

Oxford University Press is a department of the University of Oxford.
It furthers the University's objective of excellence in research, scholarship,
and education by publishing worldwide in

Oxford New York

Auckland Cape Town Dar es Salaam Hong Kong Karachi
Kuala Lumpur Madrid Melbourne Mexico City Nairobi
New Delhi Shanghai Taipei Toronto

With offices in

Argentina Austria Brazil Chile Czech Republic France Greece
Guatemala Hungary Italy Japan Poland Portugal Singapore
South Korea Switzerland Thailand Turkey Ukraine Vietnam

Oxford is a registered trade mark of Oxford University Press
in the UK and in certain other countries

Published in the United States
by Oxford University Press Inc., New York

© Oxford University Press 2009

The moral rights of the author have been asserted
Database right Oxford University Press (maker)

First published 2009

A catalogue record for this title is available from the British Library
Data available

Library of Congress Cataloguing in Publication Data
Data available

Typeset by Cepha Imaging Private Ltd., Bangalore, India
Printed in the UK by the MPG Books Group

ISBN 978–0–19–923552–0

10 9 8 7 6 5 4 3 2 1

Foreword to the second edition

It is testimony to the importance and relevance of this textbook that this new edition has been produced. Those features that made the first edition such an accessible and practical resource for general practitioners have been retained: theoretical discussion is related to the dilemmas encountered in four (fictional) practices; and the range of topics is largely the same, helping the reader to see the issues in everyday practice from cradle to grave. However, the international appeal of the book has been broadened by scattering the imaginary practices geographically, so that we now have one in Australia, one in New Zealand, one in England and one in Scotland. Writing as I now do from a medical school in Asia, perhaps I may hope for yet wider international reference in a future edition? The dilemmas of general practice are in some ways very similar worldwide, but at the same time there is no doubt that social and cultural differences set some choices in a very different light – for example, questions of the autonomy of minors and of the place of families in decision-making.

As is customary in new editions, references have been fully updated, but there are also more substantive changes, with an expansion of some of the key discussions and the clarification of others. To me, a particularly valuable change is the creation of a separate chapter discussing ethical reasoning. This contains a clear summary of the main ethical theories, but also supplies a framework for ethical reasoning and applies this to a case example. This is just the sort of practical tool that practitioners need to help them apply ethics in daily practice. (Few have the appetite or time for long philosophical disputations.) On the other hand, the authors have managed to be practical without sacrificing intellectual rigour and honesty – this book is far from being 'medical ethics for dummies'!

Things have moved on in general practice, and in medicine generally, since the first edition was published. There are now many more courses in ethics for both medical undergraduates and postgraduate trainees. Attempts have been made in Australasia, the UK and internationally through UNESCO to devise and consistently implement core curricula. It is notoriously hard to estimate the effectiveness of these educational initiatives, though it is a heartening sign that papers evaluating ethics training have become a regular feature in journals like *The Journal of Medical Ethics*, *Medical Education* and *Medical Teacher*. At the same time, maintaining ethical standards in medical practice has become even more challenging than it was when this book was first written. Despite the alleged professional commitment to putting patients first, finance seems to dominate more and more, whether it be in terms of contractual arrangements for GPs, or methods of financing and prioritizing health care services. The rush to the goldfields of 'aesthetic medicine', by GPs and specialists alike, is but one sign that equitable health care in the public sector is going to be increasingly hard to achieve. In these difficult times, one must surely wish success to this new edition, in which, as in the first edition, the practical qualities of the good general practitioner are quietly and effectively portrayed: trustworthiness, thoughtfulness, patience, generosity and integrity. These virtues are the essence of professionalism and they are what every patient wants in the inevitable medical encounters of one's life.

Alastair V. Campbell
Chen Su Lan Centennial Professor of Medical Ethics,
Yong Loo Lin School of Medicine,
National University of Singapore

Foreword to the first edition

Twenty years ago, Roger Higgs and I wrote a short book entitled, *In that case: medical ethics in everyday practice*[1]. In it, we expressed the hope that medical ethics would abandon its obsession with the dramas of hospital medicine, and begin to show the relevance of ethics to every facet of medical practice. To illustrate this, we told the story of a fictional patient, "Angie", tracing her odyssey through medical and social agencies to an ending, which may not have been ideal, but which was meant to reflect the continuing moral uncertainty of real life, and, in that, the centrality of trust.

It is refreshing to discover a new book, all these years later, which locates itself firmly in such day-to-day experiences of patients and their general practitioners, and which recognizes the special features of the relationship that general practice makes possible: a relationship with the whole patient, not just a cluster of symptoms; which potentially extends over years; and which recognizes the family and social setting of the patient. Of course, such a richness of relationship is an ideal of general practice, which cannot always be fulfilled. Patterns of practice are changing, as governments seek to influence the way that health care is delivered, and as practitioners rightly seek to protect their personal and family lives. Increasingly, practitioners may rely on the data on their computer screen to understand the full history of a patient, since group practice arrangements often mean that the patient is seen by a series of doctors. Home visits are becoming much less common, and the increasing use of after-hours on-call services often means that the person seeing the patient in an emergency is not their usual daytime practitioner. Despite these changes, the concept of a generalist or family practitioner, seeing the patient in non-emergency situations in the community, remains the pivotal point for any effective health service. Without it, the ideal of whole-person care will be lost, and the vital importance of preventive medicine and early intervention will be overlooked. We need everyday medical practice and, with it, everyday ethics.

This book offers itself as an easily accessible resource for such ethics. It should sit on the shelf of every doctor's consulting room, alongside the manuals of therapeutics and prescription. In the midst of the pressured life of

---

[1] Campbell, A. V. and Higgs, R. (1982). *In that case: medical ethics in eveyday practice.* Darton, Longman and Todd, London.

modern general practice, Wendy Rogers and Annette Braunack-Mayer provide a haven of good sense and practicality. They tease out the common ethical dilemmas of daily practice from a set of fictional vignettes of encounters with patients, which will be instantly recognizable to all practitioners. They are not afraid to provide some answers, as well as raising questions (the favoured activity of philosophers), but there is no "dumbing down" in this book, no dodging of the real complexities and uncertainties of some of the dilemmas patients and practitioners face. Each chapter offers a set of references for further reading into some issues, and the book concludes with a useful guide to the scholarly resources in medical ethics that are currently available.

Arguably, the most important part of the whole book is the closing chapter, 'On being a good doctor'. With its account of virtue ethics, this chapter emphasizes what patients have always known. We need doctors who keep up to date with their knowledge and skills and who remain scientifically active and innovative in the management of their practice. We need doctors who recognize the ethical and legal complexities of the wide range of situations they have to deal with. But beyond this, we need doctors with integrity and compassion. In medicine, as in other professions where one's personal life is exposed and trust is essential, it is the singer, not just the song that matters.

Alastair V. Campbell
Professor of Ethics in Medicine
University of Bristol
Bristol

Preface

The original edition of *Practical Ethics for General Practice* aimed to provide an account of ethics in general practice, written in a way that would be useful for practitioners, students and teachers alike. In this second edition, we are building upon that aim. We have made a number of significant changes in this edition. First, we have broadened the international scope of the book. In the original edition, we based our account of ethics upon a British model of general practice, making reference, where relevant, to UK law. For this edition, we address general practice more broadly; this revised edition will be relevant in all countries where general practitioners provide comprehensive, continuing primary care and have a gatekeeper role. This has led to changes in the location of two of the practices and fewer specific references to the law. The second major change is a new chapter on ethical reasoning and the introduction of our Practical Ethics Analysis Framework. We hope that this will be a useful resource for developing a reasoned and justified response to ethical dilemmas in practice. There is a new chapter on difficult relationships with patients that includes revised material previously included in the chapter on trust. The care of children raises a range of ethical issues; in recognition of this we have written a new chapter focusing on children. Finally, the chapter on conflicts of interest has been expanded to deal more comprehensively with the conflicts that arise in practice due to the increasing complexity of health systems organization and the lives of general practitioners. All of the original chapters have been retained and updated.

We are indebted to a number of people that have helped us with this endeavour. First, our students have provided ongoing identification and discussion of ethical issues in practice. Wendy Rogers has been using the Practical Ethics Analysis Framework in teaching at Flinders University for a number of years. This experience has been invaluable in refining the Framework for publication. Her teaching has benefitted greatly from input from colleagues in the Department of Paediatrics at Flinders University and her assistant markers, especially Cheryl Wilson. Second, Annette Braunack-Mayer revised some material while a Visiting Scholar at the Department of Ethics, Philosophy and History of Medicine at University Medical Centre, Radboud University in Nijmegen, the Netherlands. She is grateful to colleagues there and in the Departments of General Practice and Public Health at UMC for many challenging and helpful conversations. The University of Adelaide again provided generous support for her time in the Netherlands. Finally we would like to thank Ling Lee for research assistance, and our families for ongoing support and love.

Contents

List of abbreviations

BMA	British Medical Association		NHS	National Health Service
EBM	evidence-based medicine		NICE	National Institute of Health and Clinical Excellence
CADTH	Canadian Agency for Drugs and Technologies in Health		PAS	physician-assisted suicide
CAMs	complementary and alternative medications		PBAC	Pharmaceutical Benefits Advisory Committee
GMC	General Medical Council		QALY	quality adjusted life year
GP	general practitioner		RCGP	Royal College of General Practitioners
GPC	General Practitioners Committee		SARS	severe acute respiratory syndrome
HF&EA	Human Fertilization and Embryology Act		ScHARR	School of Health and Related Research
IV	intravenous		WHO	World Health Organization
IVF	*in vitro* fertilsation		WMA	World Medical Association
MSAC	Medical Services Advisory Committee			
MIDIRS	Midwives Information and Resource Service			

Introduction

General practice is at the heart of health services around the world. GPs are the point of first contact for patients, and the conduit through which other forms of medical care may be accessed. They have multiple obligations—to patients in their care, to government for responsible use of resources, to communities for the standard of health services provided. Ethics is also at the heart of health services because ethics deals with fundamental questions about what ought to be valued, including health and health services, and why we ought to value particular things. In this book we bring together these two 'hearts' in a textbook on practical ethics for general practitioners.

This book has three main aims. First, we wish to help GPs appreciate the ethically significant nature of general practice, and to draw attention to the ethical complexity of apparently mundane and everyday experience. Many of the issues and cases we discuss will be familiar to GPs and, in some cases, they may appear to raise little of ethical importance at all. We want, first and foremost, to raise awareness of the fact that ethics pervades all areas of general practice.

Second, we want to present a thoughtful and thought-provoking account of the moral foundations of general practice. In recent years there have been a number of texts published on the philosophy of medicine (Pellegrino and Thomasma 1981; Veatch 1981). While these texts identify and analyse a number of key concepts for ethical practice, their need to cover the breadth of medical practice does not allow them to focus on how these concepts are worked out in specific settings. In this book we explore the ways in which moral concepts such as trust, beneficence, respect for autonomy and fairness take on particular meanings in the general practice setting.

Our intentions in this book are not only philosophical. Our final aim is to discuss some specific ethical issues in detail, with a view to offering solutions that are practical, as well as ethically sound. Ethical analysis is occasionally accused of being too abstract and abstruse to be of much value in the real world of messy problems and difficult decisions. Contrary to this view, we want to show how moral concepts and arguments can illuminate murky situations, thus providing a way forward or clarifying a response. To this end, we have developed a framework for practical ethical analysis.

Practical ethics for general practice (2nd edn) is primarily written for GPs, GP registrars and students. With this audience in mind, we have tried to ground our description and analysis of ethical concepts in the everyday reality of general practice. Generally, our approach is to introduce a topic with cases, and to define and conceptualize moral concepts in the context of these examples. One of the difficulties with a case-oriented approach to ethics is that the cases can become too 'thin', offering too little detail and losing the charm of realism (Davis 1991). 'Thick' cases, by contrast, provide rich and full descriptions of the detail of cases, but do so at the risk of invading the privacy of individuals who constitute the case. We have attempted to guard against these twin difficulties by drawing our cases from our own experiences and the experiences of our colleagues and friends. Many of the cases had their origins in real life; however, all cases have been fictionalized in terms of people, places and events to protect privacy. Our cases are set in four imaginary general practices, with the same GPs, and sometimes the same patients, reappearing in a number of chapters. We hope this way to paint a more detailed picture of the GP and his or her work, so that, by the end of the book, the reader has some feel for what these GPs value and how they routinely approach moral problems in their work. We introduce our GPs in the following paragraphs.

The GPs and their practices

The Hackney Road Practice, London, United Kingdom: Dr Jeremy Chu and Dr Malcolm Carter

The Hackney Road Practice is a large, modern practice in an inner suburb of London. The neat and well-kept exterior of the practice is a contrast to the poverty and deprivation that surrounds it, for the practice serves a particularly poor and underprivileged community with a high proportion of immigrants from African and South-East Asian countries.

The Hackney Road practice has five GPs working in it, but our attention centres on Dr Jeremy Chu and Dr Malcolm Carter, both in their late 30s, who have been in practice here for 10 years. With 25% of his patients HIV positive, Dr Chu has developed an interest in HIV medicine, particularly in the management of AIDS in primary care settings. Over time, he has assembled a team of nurses, health visitors, psychologists and social workers with expertise in this area. Dr Carter has no special interests. He enjoys general practice, but thinks he would be just as happy in any number of other occupations. Generally, the partners get along well, although there are, as we shall see, occasional differences of opinion as to how the practice should be run.

The Wilford Practice, Wilford, Lower Flinders Ranges, Australia: Dr Jack Day and Dr Mira Singh

The Wilford Practice is the only practice in Wilford, a small town in rural South Australia. Dr Jack Day has been here for 25 years now, and he and his wife, Joan, are absolutely committed to the town and the practice. Over the years, Dr Day has had a series of assistants. Few stay more than a few years; his last assistant recently moved on and Dr Mira Singh has just joined the practice. This is Dr Singh's first position since completing her general practice training in Adelaide. She expects to enjoy the work, but she is apprehensive about the relative isolation of Wilford.

The Adelaide Road Practice, Milton, Lower Flinders Ranges, Australia: Dr Jenny Morrow

The Adelaide Road Practice is located in Milton, a town about half an hour's drive from Wilford. The practice has three doctors, of whom we will meet only one, Dr Jenny Morrow, in this book. Dr Morrow has worked at the Adelaide Road Practice since she moved into the area 18 years ago to marry a local farmer. She and her husband are close friends of Jack and Joan Day.

The St Andrew's Practice, Dunedin, New Zealand: Dr David Mackenzie, Dr John Buchan and Dr Amy Walker

The St Andrew's practice is located in central Dunedin, in an attractively renovated Victorian building. The senior partners, Dr David Mackenzie and Dr John Buchan have built the practice up, over a number of years, to be a certified teaching practice with links to the local medical school. Recently the practice took on Dr Amy Walker who, as the mother of two young children, chooses to work part time. The practice also employs a nurse. For after-hours care, the practice uses the Urgent Doctors and Accident Centre.

The Gordon Road Surgery, Glasgow, Scotland: Dr Fiona McDonald and Dr David Grainger

The Gordon Road Surgery is a large group practice in outer Glasgow. It has six GPs, including two we will meet in this book. Dr Fiona McDonald, a native Glaswegian, is in her early 40s. She has been at Gordon Road for 15 years, and she has a particular interest in women's health. Dr David Grainger has only been with the practice for 3 years. Now in his early 50s, his career path has been rather unusual, beginning with a science degree, a PhD in physics and research work, and followed by his return to study medicine in his late 30s.

The final GP character in our book is Dr Martin Schroeder. Dr Schroeder originally trained in Berlin, and has worked in Britain for 5 years now, mainly as a locum. He enjoys locum work, as it provides the flexibility that allows him to travel regularly.

Practical ethics for general practice (2nd edn) is organized around a number of key ethical concepts. We begin with a discussion, in the first two chapters, of the distinguishing features of general practice, its ethical complexities and the role of ethics and ethical theory in this milieu. A detailed case analysis in Chapter 2 is used to demonstrate our practical ethical analysis framework. In Chapter 3, we turn to an analysis of the doctor–patient relationship and explore the centrality of trust to that relationship. Trust comes more readily in relationships that develop smoothly; however, this is not always the case in general practice. Chapter 4 explores the ethical issues raised by difficult relationships between doctors and patients.

The promise of confidentiality is one of the ways that GPs make trust explicit. Chapter 5 builds on our discussion of trust with an account of the meaning, importance and limits to confidentiality.

The obligation to act beneficently—for the good of patients—is central to ethical general practice. However, working out what we mean by the good of the patient, treading the fine line between beneficent and paternalistic actions, and defining the place of evidence in good medical practice, are all issues for the GP who would be beneficent. We explore the concept of beneficence and its extent and limitations in Chapter 6.

The private face of beneficence is in the consulting room, as GP and patient meet together. The public face is more often found in debates and discussion about resource allocation. Chapter 7 explores the issues associated with allocating resources fairly in a general practice setting. We begin with a definition of resource allocation and a description of the ways in which resources are currently allocated in health systems. This is followed by an account of theories and principles for the fair distribution of resources in general practice.

In Chapter 8 we return to ethical issues that arise mainly in the context of the relationship between GP and patient with a discussion of autonomy and decision-making in general practice. We examine the meaning and importance of autonomy, the nature of informed consent, some limits to autonomy and the relationship between autonomy and responsibility.

Looking after patients at particular stages in the life cycle raises specific issues. In Chapters 9, 10 and 11, we examine ethical issues that arise at the beginning of life and in the care of pregnant women (Chapter 9), in the care of children (Chapter 10) and in care at the end of life (Chapter 11). In each chapter we draw on principles and theories that have been laid out in preceding chapters, considering the ways in which trust, respect for patient decision-making and considering the best interests of those involved can shape choices and practices at these stages of life.

Chapters 4 to 11 are principally about the ethical issues that arise out of GPs' relationships with patients. Yet many aspects of GPs' work are not undertaken directly with patients. On a daily basis, GPs interact with patients' families, doctors and other healthcare professionals, students, industry representatives, government officials and their own families. In Chapter 12 we explore the ethical issues that arise out of GPs' multiple obligations, using the concept of conflicts of interest.

In the final chapter we revisit the issues we flagged in Chapter 1—'what is general practice?' and 'what is ethically significant about general practice?'. We discuss the idea of being a good general practitioner, and we draw on insights from virtue theory to integrate motives and character into our account of ethical experience in general practice.

This brief description of the content of *Practical ethics for general practice* (2nd edn) provides an indication not only of what the book is about, but also of what it is not about. First, we are not driven by an allegiance to any particular school of philosophical thought, and we would regard ourselves as philosophically eclectic. We have not set out to prepare an ethics workbook for general practitioners, although we hope that GP trainers, GPs and students will all use the book in both formal and informal education. Nor have we been concerned specifically to develop a philosophy of general practice, although there are elements in the book that point in this direction. Finally, *Practical ethics for general practice* is not a medico-legal textbook or a code of professional conduct, although there is obviously considerable overlap between the requirements and constraints imposed by the law and professional codes and the ethical practice of medicine. Instead, we have tried to focus attention on the contribution that ethics and ethical reasoning can make to good practice. We hope that this book will provide the impetus for much good discussion, learning and activity in general practice.

References

Davis DS (1991). Rich cases. The ethics of thick description. *Hastings Center Report* **21**, 12–17.

Pellegrino ED and Thomasma DC (1981). *A philosophical basis of medicine practice*. Oxford University Press, New York.

Veatch RM (1981). *A theory of medical ethics*. Basic Books, New York.

Chapter 1

General practice and ethics

Introduction

> The generalist cannot take refuge in the limitations of his specialty. For him the healing relationship must be entered in the fullest sense.... He must help, care for, comfort and ease when the specialist has nothing to offer.... The patient often has made the rounds of the specialties; he is still ill, still needing answers to the key clinical questions. Even if the patient's illness has been 'negotiated' out of medicine by other physicians, someone must remain who can help.
>
> The generalist, on this view, is the physician par excellence since he has the most intimate relationship with the healing and helping functions of medicine. A specialist, especially if his domain is a technique, might get away with only scientifically right decisions; but a generalist, never.

(Pellegrino 1983, p.166)

> General practitioners/family doctors are specialist physicians trained in the principles of the discipline. They are personal doctors, primarily responsible for the provision of comprehensive and continuing care to every individual seeking medical care irrespective of age, sex and illness. They care for individuals in the context of their family, their community, and their culture, always respecting the autonomy of their patients. They recognise they will also have a professional responsibility to their community. In negotiating management plans with their patients they integrate physical, psychological, social, cultural and existential factors, utilising the knowledge and trust engendered by repeated contacts. General practitioners/family physicians exercise their professional role by promoting health, preventing disease and providing cure, care, or palliation. This is done either directly or through the services of others according to health needs and the resources available within the community they serve, assisting patients where necessary in accessing these services. They must take the responsibility for developing and maintaining their skills, personal balance and values as a basis for effective and safe patient care.

(WONCA Europe 2005, p.7)

General practice occupies a unique place within medicine. In many countries, it lies at the heart of the health system as one of the first points of access for anyone seeking medical care, and as the route to specialist or hospital care. In some countries, such as the United Kingdom and the Netherlands, universal registration with general practitioners formalizes this first point of contact role; in other countries, such as Australia, where there is no universal registration and patients may choose to see more than one general practitioner, the GP still functions as the conduit for access to other healthcare services.

As a discipline, general practice is relatively young; its professional colleges and academic departments formed in the 1950s and 1960s. Since then, there has been increasing attention turned towards the nature of general practice, focusing on clinical methods, philosophy and research (McWhinney 1997; Starfield 1998; Olesen *et al.* 2000; WONCA Europe 2005). Despite the difficulties of defining general practice, there are a number of points of agreement about the features that distinguish general practice from other branches of medicine. In this chapter, we briefly discuss some of the central features of general practice, and examine their ethical implications.

The GP–patient relationship

The relationship between GP and patients is a central distinguishing feature of general practice. Pellegrino draws our attention to this relationship in the quote above: in his words the relationship must be 'entered in the fullest sense', from the beginning of the patient's problems through to the exit of the last specialist. The WONCA Europe definition of general practice similarly foregrounds this relationship by emphasizing that general practitioners are 'personal doctors'. The commitment to the patient as a person is prior to any particular health problem that the patient may have. Once a patient appears at a GP's surgery, the GP is committed to providing care to that person, whether they attend the surgery frequently or infrequently, in good or ill health.

The centrality of the relationship leads directly to many of the other defining features of general practice. The commitment to the patient as a person, irrespective of their state of health, requires a holistic approach to patient care. This may be described in terms of the biopsychosocial model of health, often approached in practice through patient-centred techniques. The main point is that general practice prides itself on seeing its patients first as people, with hopes, fears, lives, jobs, families and relationships, over and above any health problem that may be presented at the surgery. Specialists may rely on their adeptness at various techniques and fulfil their medical obligations to patients with little interest in, or knowledge of, their patients' lives, but for general practice, the person comes before the disease. An ophthalmologist, for example, can effectively treat an acute penetrating eye injury in a female patient without knowing much about the patient or her life, discharging her once the injury is stable. For her GP, that injury may be one more in a succession of domestic 'accidents', but maybe this is the injury that will lead to disclosure about her violent partner and provide the opportunity for the GP to offer help that will be accepted on this occasion.

This commitment can be a double-edged sword. On one hand, knowing and understanding the circumstances of one's patients can help both diagnostically and therapeutically.

Case 1.1

Ms Jackie Silvers is a 35-year-old mother of three young children. She lives with her husband who is an executive with a computer company and who spends a lot of time away from home. Their youngest child has severe asthma, and the middle child has extremely aggressive behaviour that has responded only poorly to a series of appointments with a psychologist. Ms Silvers presents on this occasion with recurrent headaches. Dr Buchan knows that her husband is away in the USA on a three-week trip, and that the youngest child was admitted last week as an emergency with his asthma. Ms Silvers has recently had a promotion in her work and is now managing a team of staff in the local council offices.

Dr Buchan takes a history and examines Ms Silvers. His provisional diagnosis is that these are tension headaches, exacerbated by recent stresses in Ms Silvers' life.

In this case, Dr Buchan's knowledge of Ms Silvers as a person, coupled with a thorough history and examination, help him to reach a diagnosis and to spare Ms Silvers the inconvenience and anxiety of further investigations. He is able to help by explaining the likely association between the headaches and her current situation, and suggest practical ways for Ms Silvers to manage her own stress and the children's problems.

Sometimes, however, the commitment to a holistic approach and to the patient as a person can be challenging, especially when that person follows a course of action that we do not agree with or, like the victim of domestic violence, is unable to acknowledge the real problem or accept help. In these cases, the GP cannot walk away from the relationship, but is committed to offering whatever care can be negotiated with the patient at that moment in time. The frustrations of missed opportunities, ongoing damage to health and limited scope for action can be demoralizing.

This leads us to the next feature of the GP–patient relationship: it continues over time, rather than being limited to discrete illnesses. Whether the GP is the sole provider of care, or shares his contact over time with other health professionals, this continuity itself feeds into the relationship, as it allows GPs to know their patients in sickness and in health. The prostrate figure lying vomiting in a dark room with a migraine headache may on another day be a cheerful and confident gardener who has come in for a tetanus injection. Episodic care over time allows both GP and patient to build up their knowledge of each other and, as we discuss in chapter 3, this is fundamental to the growth of trust in the relationship. Again, the ongoing nature of the relationship can be both rewarding and challenging. Looking after pregnant women and later their children, or following up a patient after a serious illness are some of the joys of ongoing care. On the other hand, the prospect of years of appointments with patients who have problems that seem insoluble can be daunting.

The comprehensive nature of general practice means that for GPs, surprise is a constant companion. Patients may present with something as routine as an upper respiratory tract infection, or as rare as vacation-acquired tropical disease. The tension headaches may become sinister in nature, or the recurrent complaint of tiredness be due to anaemia rather than depression. Problems may be physical, psychological or social; they may be amenable or refractory to diagnosis and there may or may not be something that the GP can do about them. Whatever problems patients bring to their GPs, a response is required; the GP is expected to do something. Even if the patient does not present with a problem, the GP is expected to carry out preventive care.

As well as relationships with individual patients, GPs may also have relationships with families. Of course, not all members of a family necessarily attend the same practice, but often a GP will see more than one family member in her practice. Again, this can be helpful in terms of understanding the person who is the patient on this occasion, and the way that the illness is likely to impact upon both the family and the person.

There are three final features about general practice that affect the GP–patient relationship. The first is the location of general practice, in the community in small self-contained surgeries. In comparison with hospitals, general practice surgeries are less intimidating and offer a greater promise of intimacy. Surgeries are often close to people's homes, so that there can be a shared knowledge and understanding of the community. The GP will know if there is adequate (or any) public transport, or if the local factory or school is closing down. Consultations may take place in the patient's home, providing GPs with sometimes invaluable insights into the lives of their patients. This proximity between the medical and the domestic spheres is rare in other branches of medicine.

The GP's familiarity with the local community also creates opportunities for GPs to provide care to whole communities. For example, the GP whose practice is situated in a suburb with a high proportion of refugee immigrants may acquire a role as advocate for health and social services targeted to the needs of this group. Or, close proximity to a mine may give the GP opportunities to participate in health-promotion campaigns for all mine workers, not just those who regularly attend her surgery. The GP may also be called upon to be the agent of government in delivering public health services to the community or in monitoring the health status of the community.

Finally, general practice is usually the first point of access for patients seeking medical care. Some patients present straight to hospital with emergencies, some use drop-in centres or seek advice from pharmacists but, for most patients, it is a visit to the GP that heralds any episode of healthcare. This means that GPs become familiar with the full range of symptoms that trigger a visit to the doctor, as well as becoming familiar with the variations in threshold that lead some patients to consult only when *in extremis*, while other consult more readily. If a problem is beyond the expertise of the GP, or if further tests or therapies are required, it is the GP who acts as gatekeeper to secondary and tertiary care. Even in health systems that do not accord the GP a gatekeeper role, GPs still play a role in helping patients choose and obtain the most appropriate care (Olesen *et al.* 2000). And it is to the GP that the patient returns after colleagues in other specialties have made their contributions to the patient's care.

Ethical complexities in general practice

What are the ethical implications of the features of general practice that we have outlined above? Perhaps the most significant feature is that general practice is ethically complex. The GP–patient relationship means that GPs are often closer to their patients and their patients' lives than doctors working in other medical specialities. The closeness of this relationship can lead to insights into ethical values that would not be obvious in other settings. One of the central debates in medical ethics concerns finding the right balance between acting for the good of the patient and respecting patient's rights to self-determination (Christie and Hoffmaster 1986). The ethical terms for these two values are beneficence and respect for autonomy. Historically, acting for the good of the patient has been the dominant value in medicine. Over the past 50 years this has changed, with recognition of the rights of patients to have a much greater say in their treatment. In many branches of medicine, there can be a quite stark demarcation between these values, with the medical view of what is good for the patient competing with the patient's own view of what is good for them. In general practice, there is far more opportunity to know the patient as a person above and beyond their illness, so that the medical view about the right thing to do becomes influenced by the GP's knowledge of the patient and what is important to them. We pick up this issue in detail in Chapter 6.

GPs' views about the autonomy of their patients are also influenced by their personal knowledge about their patients' lives and circumstances. Rather than having to make an assessment of the patient's capacity for self-determination at one point in time (for example, in hospital before an operation or in a rushed out-patient clinic appointment), GPs are able to form a detailed picture of their patients' lives and develop a greater understanding of the ways that their circumstances influence the choices that they are able to make. The traditional medical ethics view of respecting autonomy is that if patients are fully informed, have a good understanding of the information necessary to make a decision and are not coerced, then any decision they make is autonomous and should be respected by the doctor (patient autonomy is discussed in detail in Chapter 8). But for general practice, this seems unduly narrow. GPs are able to assess the wider context and to look for factors in their patients' lives that might shape the decisions that seem possible (Doyal 1999). A doctor in an out-patient clinic might accept an elderly woman's decision to refuse an operation for a hip replacement as an autonomous decision, as long as the patient is informed and understands the implications of her decision. For her GP, who knows that the patient is worried about who might look after her frail husband while she is in hospital and recovering from the operation, the decision might appear in a different light. Rather than accepting her decision to forego surgery, the GP would be able to use his relationship with the woman to explore the barriers to surgery, and to ensure that her decision is based upon her own preferences rather than driven by circumstances that she finds overwhelming.

Confidentiality is a key issue in medical ethics. The ethical requirements are straightforward: information about patients should not be divulged to any one else except in quite strictly regulated circumstances (these are discussed in Chapter 5). For doctors working in hospitals removed from the communities where their patients live, it is not difficult to maintain confidentiality. For GPs, who may look after multiple members of families, keeping information private can be challenging. What if one person's medical information has implications for the health of other members of the family? A woman might see her GP complaining of tiredness and difficulty coping with her elderly father whose behaviour is becoming erratic. She might think that the problems in coping with her father are due to a recurrence of her depression, which she has had in the past. The GP, however, may be aware that the father's behaviour is due to cerebral secondaries from a disseminated cancer, information that the father does not want his daughter to know. The ethical obligation to maintain confidentiality can be difficult if the GP is witness to the distress that secrecy can sometimes cause in families.

The nature of the GP–patient relationship, and the GP's role as gate-keeper to other aspects of the health service, mean that patients often rely heavily on GPs to be their advocates. This can create an open-ended commit-ment–where should GPs draw the line in advocating for their patients? For doctors in other specialities, it is possible to look after patients within the boundaries of their speciality, and to withdraw once those limits are reached. In general practice, medical problems merge into social problems. There is no clear boundary line; many problems are neither clearly within nor outside the medical domain. In addition, GPs are aware of the struggles that patients may have dealing with other health services or welfare agencies, and know that unless they help, the patient is likely to struggle unsuccessfully.

The advocacy role, together with open access to general practice, mean that GPs often face unrealistic moral demands (Doyal 1999). How can they meet the needs of their patients when there is barely enough time to see everyone who wants an appointment, when many of their patients' problems are the result of social rather than physiological processes, and when their patients are competing with other patients for scarce resources? And how can GPs be fair in their gatekeeping role while trying to be advocates for their patients?

Medical professionalism involves not just the relationship between a physi-cian and a patient, as discussed in Chapters 3 and 4, and relationships with colleagues and other health professionals, which is treated in Chapter 12, it also involves a relationship with society. This relationship can be character-ized as a 'social contract' whereby society grants the profession privileges, including exclusive or primary responsibility for the provision of certain serv-ices and a high degree of self-regulation, and in return, the profession agrees to use these privileges primarily for the benefit of others and only secondarily for its own benefit.

The social responsibilities of general practitioners create further ethical complexities. GPs may be expected to fulfil public health roles in their com-munities that do not necessarily sit easily with their commitment to individual patients. For example, the recent SARS threat has highlighted the tensions inherent in the roles GPs could play in preventing or containing an epidemic. A study conducted by Wong et al. (2004) found that GPs were reluctant to quarantine themselves or give quarantine leave to their staff during the SARS epidemic, suggesting that GPs placed a high value on caring for their own patients, even when providing care might not serve broader public health goals. GPs who treat patients they suspect of involvement in terrorism also face difficult decisions in balancing the needs of the patient in their surgery against wider community interests.

A final ethical complexity is the way that general practice is organized. The relative isolation of general practice means that opportunities for ethical discussion are limited, either because there is no-one with whom to discuss ethical issues, or there is no time to do so, given the multitude of pressures on GPs' time. This isolation can magnify ethical complexities, making dilemmas appear insoluble.

Conclusion

General practice shares various features with other branches of medicine, but the combination that occurs in general practice makes it unique. All of the features that we have mentioned in our discussions, the importance of the relationship and the comprehensive and continuing nature of care, lead to ethical complexity and raise ethical issues that are deserving of specific consideration. Making sense of these ethical issues requires tools in the identification, analysis and resolution of ethical issues. In the next chapter we turn to a discussion of ethical deliberation and its use in a general practice context.

References

Christie R and Hoffmaster B (1986). *Ethical issues in family medicine.* Oxford University Press, New York.

Doyal L (1999). Ethico-legal dilemmas within general practice, moral indeterminacy and abstract morality. In Dowrick C and Frith L (ed.) *General practice and ethics, uncertainty and responsibility.* Routledge, London.

McWhinney I (1997). *A textbook of family medicine* (2nd edn). Oxford University Press, New York.

Oakley J (2001). A virtue ethics approach. In Kuhse H and Singer P. (ed.) *A companion to bioethics.* Blackwell Publishers, Oxford, 86–97.

Olesen F, Dickinson J and Hjortdahl P (2000). General practice–time for a new definition *BMJ* **320**, 354–357.

Pellegrino E (1983). The healing relationship, the architectonics of clinical medicine. In Shelp E. (ed.) *The clinical encounter, the moral fabric of the patient-physician relationship.* D. Reidel Publishing Company, Dordrecht, 153–172.

Starfield B (1998). *Primary care, balancing health needs, services and technology.* Oxford University Press, New York.

WONCA Europe (2005). *The European definition of general practice/family medicine.* (accessed 11 December 2007) at http,//www.woncaeurope.org/

Wong WCW, Lee A, Tsang KK and Wong SYS (2004). How did general practitioners protect themselves, their family, and staff during the SARS epidemic in Hong Kong? *Journal of Epidemiology and Community Health* **58**, 180–185.

Chapter 2

Ethical reasoning and general practice

Introduction

In Chapter 1 we suggested that general practice was an 'ethically complex' activity. Just what do we mean when we say that general practice is ethically complex? What do these terms 'ethics' and 'ethical' entail? And what, if anything, does ethics and ethical analysis have to offer us as we go about our daily lives? In this chapter, we provide a brief discussion of ethical theory, describe a framework for analysing ethical problems and give an example of how the approach and theory can be used to make decisions.

The role of ethical deliberation in general practice

Broadly speaking, ethics deals with the decisions and choices that we make in our lives. The first questions in ethics often may be: what should I do in this situation, or what would a good GP do here? Often there is little doubt about how to respond to these questions and, for the most part, we don't even think about our responses. A patient hobbles in with a sprained ankle–we strap it and prescribe painkillers and rest. Another patient bursts into tears in the consulting room–we reach for the tissues and try to console her. Such responses may seem straightforward. We do not usually stop to consider why we are acting in this way, still less analyse our responses in ethical language. In much of general practice care, ethics drops out of view and we do not think something like: 'I was acting beneficently towards the patient with a sprained ankle when I treated her'.

Sometimes, however, there can be doubt about how to respond. Should I hospitalize this patient with end-stage renal failure? Should I push this wavering mother, so that she will decide to have her children vaccinated today? What are my responsibilities when a patient's family thinks I am doing the wrong thing for their relative? What do I do when a patient asks me to do something I don't want to do? In these situations our confusion may arise because we can envisage more than one appropriate action, or because no action seems quite right.

In both the clear and the confusing cases, ethical deliberation involves further questions that try to uncover our reasons and the values that lie behind those reasons. *Why* should I help someone with a sprained ankle? Because I have the skills to help and my treatment will stop the patient from suffering pain, and help to restore them to good health. We can take the questions further: why is it good to reduce suffering, and why do we think that health is so important? The role of ethics is to uncover the reasons that lie behind our assumptions and habits, and to analyse these reasons through a moral lens. This can help us to fashion systematic ways to respond to the choices we face. Ethical reflection provides a way to clarify our values, and to impose some consistency on the confusion of our moral lives.

Ultimately the ethical question is always a 'why' question, for two reasons. First, ethics has an important role in making explicit the taken-for-granted assumptions that underpin our actions. Reflecting on mundane and routine decisions helps us to identify the values guiding our decisions, and allows us the opportunity to reconsider these. Second, ethical reasoning is most often invoked when we cannot see a straightforward answer to the question, What is the right thing to do? If we do not know what the best choice is in a situation, it seems fairly obvious that we then examine why certain choices might be better or worse than others, and look at the deeper values that lead us to those judgments.

Because ethics usually surfaces in medical discussions when doctors are faced with an ethically difficult decision and want to know what to do, ethical deliberation can be a very frustrating exercise. Doctors often want specific answers to specific problems, but ethics and ethical reasoning will not always provide an answer for each unique and individual situation. There is no medical ethics rule book that will identify the right thing to do. What ethical debate and deliberation can offer are ways of thinking about problems, ways of identifying the values that may be in conflict and ways of systematically clarifying issues.

Ethical theory

In this book, we base many of our discussions around cases, and we discuss the ethically relevant features in relation to the cases. In our discussions, we draw upon three standard approaches to ethical analysis. These involve looking at the consequences of different courses of action, looking at the duties or obligations of those making the decisions, and looking at the character and virtues of the decision-maker. In ethical terms, these three approaches are called consequentialism, deontology and virtue ethics.

Consequentialism

As its name suggests, consequentialism is the view that it is the consequences of actions that determine their morality. This is an appealing view, as it links morality to the effects of our actions. Most of us intuitively consider the consequences of actions when we think about the goodness or badness of those actions. This is particularly so in medicine, where we rely upon the good consequences of our actions to help patients. Why is it good to remove an infected appendix? Because this restores the patient to health; the operation has beneficial consequences. It is belief in the good consequences of our actions that lies behind our therapeutic interventions.

The most famous consequentialist theory is utilitarianism, which links consequences with maximizing welfare or happiness. Many people are familiar with the utilitarian saying 'the greatest good for the greatest number'. Utilitarians believe that the consequences of actions are morally important, so far as they affect the welfare or happiness of people. Actions that promote welfare are morally preferable to those that do not promote welfare. In addition, actions that maximize welfare are morally preferable to those that do not maximize welfare.

How does this work in practice? Utilitarianism requires working out which consequences matter and to whom. The welfare of each person affected by the action must be considered in the calculation, with each person counting for one and no-one counting for more than one (Hare 2001; Häyry 2007). So if we have an action, for example, prescribing antibiotics for a woman with a urinary tract infection, there will be a good consequence for the patient in terms of her welfare, and we do not anticipate any ill consequences. The action seems morally worthy. Should we consider anyone else in the calculation? Probably not in normal circumstances. But if the woman had to be seen as an emergency in preference to another patient with severe back pain, or if there were a shortage of antibiotics, so that her treatment precluded treatment for a child with pneumonia, then we would have to include the harms to those other people in our calculation. It is in the practical details that utilitarianism and consequentialism become difficult. Utilitarianism requires assigning a value to each consequence. But how do you give a certain state of affairs a value? One approach is to focus on people's preferences or the satisfaction of their wants and desires. The utilitarian using this approach attempts to find out what people would prefer to do when they have a range of possible choices, takes account of how strongly they feel about their choices and tries to ensure that as many preferences are fulfilled as possible. Despite the apparent simplicity of this approach, assigning a value to outcomes is notoriously difficult.

How do we weigh up the value of a short life with cancer compared to a longer life in and out of the oncology unit for chemotherapy, or the uncertainty and risks of spinal surgery compared with the pain of a chronic disc prolapse?

Apart from these practical problems, consequentialism does not distinguish between intended and unintended consequences of actions, and yet we often believe that accidental outcomes should be judged differently from intended outcomes. If the woman prescribed with antibiotics has a severe anaphylactic reaction (despite no history of sensitivity to the drugs in question), this outcome harms her welfare. We do not, however, judge the doctor to be morally blame-worthy in the way that we would if he had set out deliberately to harm her.

Despite some of the difficulties, consequentialism plays an important role in our moral reflection. At many points in this text, we will delineate and take account of the outcomes of actions. However, we shall also consider other morally relevant factors, such as the duties of those involved, and their character and motives.

Deontological theories

Deontological theories hold that there are inherent or intrinsic features of acts that are morally significant, rather than their consequences. These theories are concerned with specifying duties in relation to acts that are either morally prohibited or required. Modern deontology is based upon the Kantian princi-ple of unconditional respect for persons. This principle requires always treat-ing others (and oneself) as ends in themselves, rather than as means to ends (Boyle 2001; McNaughton and Rawling 2007; O'Neill 2007). Following this principle gives us duties not to deceive or coerce people, as this does not treat them as ends in themselves. If a GP enrols a patient in a drug trial without telling them about the payment that the GP receives for each enrolment, the patient might benefit from the drug and be none the wiser about the GP's financial arrangements. The consequences might be very satisfactory for both patient and GP. But a deontological analysis would maintain that the GP's action was wrong, because he deceived the patient and used the patient's involvement in the trial to benefit himself.

Duty-based theories in healthcare often focus upon the duties and obliga-tions that arise out of the specific circumstances in which we live and work. In this book, we will be concerned chiefly with duties that attach to the role of general practitioner. We will explore a number of these duties in some detail—duties to keep faith with those with whom one has agreements, to pre-vent harm and promote good, to respect the autonomous choices of others, to ensure that others receive their fair due, to be trustworthy. Out of these duties grow some specific rules and practices. The duty to obtain informed consent for medical treatment, for example, is grounded in the principle that we should respect the autonomous choices of others. The duty to tell the truth and be honest in communication between doctors and patients is grounded in the obligation to avoid deception and to be trustworthy.

Just as consequentialist theories have problems, so too do duty-based theories. One difficulty is the problem of deciding on a course of action if duties seem to conflict. Based upon the principle of respect for persons, GPs should respect the autonomous choices of their patients. We have already alluded to some of the difficulties in knowing when a decision is autonomous. Apart from this, difficulties may arise if patients ask us to do something that breaches other duties. For example, the elderly man with cerebral secondaries in the example above did not want us to tell his daughter of his condition, but honouring his request involves deception towards his daughter on the GP's part. How should we weigh up obeying one duty that is in conflict with another?

Duties and consequences are morally important. Both of these approaches involve our original question 'What is the right thing to do?' and offer answers that are justified by appeals to fundamental principles or to the consequences of actions. There is a third way to approach our question, and this turns us away from judging actions, to looking at the characteristics and motivation of the person who is acting.

Virtue ethics

Virtue ethics directs our attention to particular qualities and character traits that are morally relevant. Our question about the right thing to do is answered by saying: 'The right thing to do is what a good person would do'. This approach is appealing for general practice because so much of general practice is grounded in the doctor–patient relationship, and the moral quality of the relationship depends very much upon the qualities that each person brings to it. Qualities like honesty, compassion, integrity and justice are likely to support a good relationship, while deception, laziness and greed will undermine the relationship. Virtue ethics relies upon identifying a series of virtues that are necessary for human flourishing, that is describing a set of characteristics that we accept as good (Oakley 2001, 2007). In healthcare, virtue theories link to the goals of medicine, so that beneficence is an important virtue, as are compassion and respect. Trying to do what a good GP would do in these circumstances can be a helpful action guide, particularly if we have been lucky enough to work with one or more GPs whom we admire for their wisdom in ethically challenging circumstances.

Despite these attractions, virtue theory has drawbacks. For GPs, perhaps the most important criticism is that virtue theory does not always provide guides for action: emphasizing good character does not automatically tell us what to *do* in difficult situations. Virtue theorists have responded to this challenge by describing in some detail the virtues associated with particular roles and how they apply in particular situations (Oakley 2007). We explore some of these situations in more detail, when we return to the question of the virtuous GP in the final chapter.

A framework for analysing ethical problems

The sections above on consequentialism, deontology and virtue theory give only the shortest of introductions to these rich traditions in moral theory. Even in these brief accounts, though, it should be apparent that these moral theories offer different ways to approach, explore and resolve moral dilemmas. Most people working in medical ethics develop ways in which they can use the insights these moral theories offer to inform their own analyses of ethical problems. Indeed, many introductory texts on medical ethics will include a section that outlines a framework for ethical analysis. In this section, we describe one such framework and provide an example of its use in analysing a specific ethical problem in general practice. Our practical ethics analysis framework can be used equally well to facilitate reflection on a problem that is already in the past, to guide decision-making in the present or even to imagine how one might respond to a problem that arises in the future.

It may help to think of the practical ethics framework as similar to the frameworks for history taking and examination that medical students learn in the early years of medical education. The novice finds a set pattern of questions and prompts immensely useful in their first attempts to take a history and examine a patient; in a similar way, our ethics analysis framework is designed to help practitioners to identify and to explicate the major components of an ethical problem and to use the theories outlined above in productive ways.

A useful way to begin an ethical analysis is with a *case summary*–the key features of the patient's history, including relevant clinical information. This should not be an exhaustive account of all clinical findings, investigations, medications, social factors. Rather, it should provide sufficient detail so that others can understand the relevant issues in the case. A *problem list* is also helpful at this point; a short list of the ethical, legal and social or cultural issues, either existing or anticipated, is a way to clarify exactly what the issues are and what kind of issues they are. Although ethical, legal, social and cultural issues will often overlap, it can be very constructive to make clear the differences between these issues. For example, when a GP wonders about the cause of bruising on a newborn's arms, he has both legal issues (related to his statutory obligation to report suspicion of child abuse) and ethical issues (for example, what action here will most likely secure the child's best interests) to consider.

The ethical *case analysis* proper starts with the patient, and then moves on to the practitioner and other groups affected by the case. It should begin with the *patient's perspective*, focusing on the patient's needs, wants and rights, as well as any specific cultural issues, important relationships, and other medical and non-medical factors. The *practitioner's duties and obligations* need to be articulated in terms of ethical duties, legal obligations and professional obligations, many of which we will explore in more detail in the following chapters. By this stage in the analysis, many people will have some idea about what they think the 'best' thing to do is. The analysis should consider the *consequences* of this course of action for all those whose lives are touched by the case. This can begin with the patient, but it needs also to consider the consequences for the patient's family, the GP, other members of the healthcare team, the health services that may be involved and the wider community. Discussion of potential (or actual) conflict between health professionals, damage to relationships, implications for the medical profession and considerations of the implications for other patients can all be considered here. The 'front page' test provides a useful question to ask here: what might the media say about the case if it became public? No ethical analysis is complete without canvassing *alternatives*. What other possible ways of dealing with this situation are there? Why might these alternative courses of action be ethically better or worse than what actually happened or than the first, intuitive, response?

Finally, all ethics case analyses need a *conclusion*–a clear statement of the decision or preferred course of action in relation to problems identified in the problem list. This should also include a summary of the reasons offered for the decision. A schematic outline of the practical ethics analysis framework is given in Box 2.1.

Box 2.1 Practical ethics analysis framework

1. Case Summary

A summary of the patient's history and relevant clinical information.

2. Problem list

Ethical issues: capacity to give informed consent, intra-familial care and responsibility, potential breach of confidentiality.

Legal issues: statutory obligations of medical practitioners, legal regulation of contraceptives or abortion, legal statutes in relation to end of life requests.

Social/cultural issues: differing cultural views on breaking bad news and decision-making, traditions of apparent paternalism.

3. Case analysis

Patient's perspective:

Patient's needs, wants, rights, cultural issues, medical and non-medical, relationships and so on.

Practitioner's duties and obligations:

Ethical duties (e.g. beneficence, trustworthiness, honesty, respect).

Legal obligations.

Professional obligations.

Consequences for:

Patient.

Practitioners.

Healthcare team.

Hospital.

Community.

4. Alternatives

Discuss alternative courses of action where relevant, and why these might be better or worse.

5. Conclusion

This should be a clear statement, with reasons, of the preferred course of action in relation to the ethical issues.

Using the framework: Dr Morrow and Lisa

This case analysis uses our ethical analysis framework to analyse a difficult situation which, although uncommon, should resonate with the experience of many rural GPs. Rather than following the framework slavishly point by point, we have used it as a scaffold on which ethical issues can be placed and arguments can be presented. We have also tried to convey the dynamic nature of ethical decision-making here–Dr Morrow has to make a decision 'on the run', which she then has the opportunity to revisit, ethically speaking, after the event.

Case summary

Lisa is a 15-year-old girl who lives in Milton. She comes to see her GP, Dr Morrow, to discuss contraception. Lisa has recently become sexually active with her boyfriend of 8 months. There has been no coercion, and the decision to have sex has been made together by Lisa and her boyfriend after lengthy deliberation. This is her first 'serious' boyfriend and Lisa regards it as a stable relationship. Lisa has no significant past history, is on no medication and does not smoke. She attends secondary school and lives at home with both parents and her older brother and younger sister. She is a reasonably mature and sensible girl, she does well at school, has supportive friendships, and is good at sports. Her mother is not aware of Lisa's sexual behaviour or her request for contraception.

This comparatively straightforward situation is complicated by the fact that Lisa is Dr Morrow's niece, the daughter of her husband's sister. Relationships between Dr Morrow's family and Lisa's family are close, they get on well together and they regularly see each other socially.

Dr Morrow has provided Lisa's mother and her three children with medical care for the past 12 years. The availability of female doctors in Milton has been limited over this time and Lisa's family has been happy for Dr Morrow to take this role. On this occasion Lisa has come to Dr Morrow in confidence, requesting objective and unbiased treatment.

Problem list

Ethical issues:

Respecting autonomy in a 15-year-old.

Assessing competence in a 15-year-old.

Informed consent.

Maintaining confidentiality in treatment of family members and friends.

Trust in relationships, both professional and personal.

Legal issues:

> Age of consent for medical treatment and Gillick competence.
>
> Age of consent for intercourse.

Social/cultural issues:

> Limited access to alternative medical services.
>
> Family relationships.

Case analysis

In 'real life' the patient's perspective and the practitioner's obligations are often closely related. Although this case analysis begins with Lisa's needs and wishes, it moves quickly to a discussion of Dr Morrow's obligations to meet those needs. There is an intermediate point in the analysis at which it seems clear that Dr Morrow's ethical obligation is to prescribe the contraceptive pill for Lisa. However, reviewing the consequences of this action for Dr Morrow and her wider family disturbs what has appeared a settled decision. Dr Morrow's final decision reflects a mix of all elements of reasoning in the case analysis.

The patient's perspective

The principle of respect for patients' autonomy protects the right that patients have to control their own bodies and to make their own decisions about medical treatment (see Chapter 8). Lisa, at 15, feels that she should have the right to make her own decisions about her relationships, sexual activity and healthcare. She is unaware of any legal guidelines about age of consent. In the country in which this case is set (Australia), consent for medical treatment for patients less than 18 years of age is generally provided by their parents or guardians. However, there are circumstances in which children and adolescents can consent to their treatment without their parents' knowledge. The premise of Gillick competence means that if the medical practitioner is satisfied that the person has the understanding and intelligence to enable him to understand fully the nature and implications of the proposed treatment, that person is competent to make their own decisions regardless of their age (see Chapter 10). In some states of Australia, a child under the age of 16 years can consent to medical treatment if:

1. the medical practitioner who is to administer the treatment is of the opinion that the child is capable of understanding the nature, consequences and risks of the treatment, and that the treatment is in the best interest of the child's health and well-being; and

2. that opinion is supported by the written opinion of at least one other medical practitioner who personally examines the child before the treatment is commenced.

A second important issue from Lisa's perspective is confidentiality. If a child is deemed to be Gillick competent, then she is entitled to the same standard of medical care as anyone else, including confidentiality (Chapter 10). Lisa had approached Dr Morrow as a GP and asked her to respect her privacy. As a GP this is not a problem, but as an 'Auntie' this presents a little more of a challenge! Once Dr Morrow had decided for herself that she was going to continue the consultation with her, maintaining confidentiality requires that she assure Lisa that she will keep whatever is said confidential unless she feels that to do so would put Lisa at risk of significant harm. Dr Morrow also agrees that, if she does need to tell Lisa's parents anything, she will let Lisa know first, and arrange for her to be present when her parents are informed. This strategy safeguards Lisa from the possibility of Dr Morrow informally chatting to her mother at the next family lunch.

The practitioner's duties and obligations

Dr Morrow is aware of her legal obligations and, in order to fulfil them, she discusses the implications of sexual activity with Lisa in some detail. She deals not only with the need for contraception but also with protection against sexually transmitted illness, some of the psychological and relationship implications that accompany the commencement of a sexual relationship, the risks and benefits of different types of contraception, side-effects of the oral contraceptive pill (Lisa's preferred method of contraception), and Lisa's thoughts about the possibility of an unplanned pregnancy and what she would choose to do in that situation.

After a long discussion, Dr Morrow is satisfied that Lisa is capable of understanding and does indeed understand all aspects of her decision. Put another way, she is confident that Lisa is making an informed decision. Three elements are crucial to the concept of informed consent. These are that patients need to be competent to make the decision, they must understand the necessary information, and the decision must be made freely and without coercion (Chapter 8). In discussing all of the above aspects of sexual activity and its associated health risks, and contraception, Dr Morrow is able to satisfy herself that Lisa is truly informed in her decision. Dr Morrow also feels that to provide Lisa with contraception is in the best interests of her health, as use of the contraceptive pill is of less risk to her medically and psychologically than an unplanned pregnancy. Lisa has already made the decision to become sexually active and is planning to continue in this relationship, so it is in her interests to provide her with adequate and appropriate education and resources.

At this point in the analysis, a decision to provide Lisa with a prescription for the oral contraceptive pill would be consistent with a range of ethical principles: it serves Lisa's best interests, respects her autonomy, maintains confidentiality and is likely to have good outcomes.

Other consequences

There is one issue that does not fit neatly into this summary–the appropriateness of treating family members and friends. Such conflicts of interest can influence professional judgement, as well as leading to a strain in personal relationships. Dr Morrow often treats people she knows socially, and she is familiar with trying to put aside her personal relationships with them so that she can listen and treat them objectively. She has developed some techniques to manage this ethically. Before a consultation starts, she explains her 'ground rules': if either she or her patient is uncomfortable–if one of them feels that the personal relationship is affecting the medical relationship or, alternatively, if the medical relationship is compromising the personal friendship–then this needs to be discussed and other arrangements for treating the patient need to be made. Dr Morrow discusses these issues briefly with Lisa, who decides she still wants Dr Morrow to continue in the role of her GP.

Trust is an important part of any doctor–patient relationship, especially in general practice. It is equally important in family relationships and friendships. Lisa came to Dr Morrow as her GP because she felt that she could trust her in that role. Lisa also trusts Dr Morrow as her aunt to respect this relationship. However, Lisa is perhaps ignorant of Dr Morrow's need to maintain and be trustworthy in her relationship with her sister-in-law. Dr Morrow wants and needs to respect Lisa's autonomy and confidentiality as a GP; however, as her mother's sister-in-law she did not want to be seen to be keeping secrets or colluding with behaviour that her sister-in-law may not agree with. There is an ethical 'cost' for Dr Morrow in this situation that she can not share with Lisa.

For Dr Morrow, it is the dilemma of respecting Lisa's trust and providing her with good medical treatment, while also maintaining her relationship with the rest of the family, that is the most troubling. Ultimately, Dr Morrow decides that she will not be able to prescribe contraception to Lisa and that she will need to help Lisa make other arrangements. In conveying this to Lisa the conversation takes a surprising turn: Lisa is actually quite amenable to the suggestion that she discuss both her sexual relationship and her request for contraception with her mother. Eventually Dr Morrow gives Lisa a prescription for the combined oral contraceptive pill, and Lisa agrees to go home and discuss this with her mother before filling the script.

Alternatives

Providing contraception to a sexually active 15-year-old is a relatively common general practice activity, and although the guidelines for underage medical treatment and consent are clear, there are several alternatives. Some GPs may choose not to provide contraception, insisting on parental consent, thereby running the risk of ignoring patient autonomy in favour of other factors. Some may decide to inform the young woman about the medical consequences of her behaviour, not inform her parents, but not provide contraception. Many others would write out the script without even thinking about her age, respecting autonomy, but not taking full account of the patient's medical needs or likely consequences for her sexual behaviour, her use of contraception, and her future relationships with the medical profession. None of these strategies seem particularly satisfactory. Leaving aside the complications raised by the fact that Lisa is Dr Morrow's niece, Dr Morrow's initial decision–to provide Lisa with a prescription for the oral contraceptive pill–is the most acceptable.

The fundamental issue here, however, is really the appropriateness of treating family members in this situation, and of trust in relationships. Lisa seems ignorant of the dilemma she has created for Dr Morrow, thinking only of her need for an understanding doctor. The problem reflects a difficult aspect of 'being a professional': the need to behave so that patients remain unaware of the dilemmas they unwittingly create. In hindsight, perhaps Dr Morrow should have foreseen such situations and addressed the issue earlier by requesting that Lisa's family find another GP. Alternatively, she could have stopped Lisa's consultation as soon as she realised what she wanted, explained her reasons and asked her to make an appointment to see another GP. However, it had probably taken Lisa a lot of courage to come to Dr Morrow in the first place; sending her away may have jeopardised their personal relationship, and Dr Morrow could not have been absolutely confident that Lisa would have made an appointment with someone else.

Conclusion

Given that Lisa agreed to involve her mother, the course of action taken was probably the most ethically acceptable. Lisa received medical advice, education regarding her sexual health and appropriate contraception from her doctor of choice. Lisa's mother was informed later in the process, but appreciated the honest discussion she then had with her daughter. Dr Morrow was able to fulfil her responsibility as a GP, while maintaining both Lisa's trust in her and her relationship with Lisa's family.

If Lisa had not been so compliant and agreed to involving her mother, the situation might have ended quite differently. Dr Morrow would have been in a much more difficult position: legally she should have either involved another doctor or gained consent from Lisa's parent prior to writing out the prescription for contraception. Her decision turned, to a great degree, on the trust that she felt Lisa deserved after their honest discussion together; she felt she could be confident that Lisa would carry out her agreement to talk with her mother after the consultation.

Postscript

Dr Morrow received a grateful phone call from Lisa's mother later that week thanking her for her assistance, relieved that her daughter had sought help and informing her that Lisa had indeed talked about (most of!) what she had told Dr Morrow. Of course, she then had to let her sister-in-law know that she could not discuss any aspects of the situation with her due to her duty of confidentiality to Lisa!

Conclusion

We began this chapter by suggesting that ethical deliberation is of value in both straightforward and troubling situations. Its utility can be enhanced by making judicious use of theory and by developing and using a framework for analysis. In our case discussions in the following chapters, we pick up on all three approaches to ethical analysis that we have discussed here and we use different aspects of our analysis framework. Sometimes, situations will seem to lend themselves more to one sort of reasoning than another. At other times, one or other perspective will provide an appropriate corrective to an unbalanced analysis. What is central to our interpretation of ethics in general practice is the relationship between doctor and patient. This is explored in depth in the next chapter.

References

Boyle J (2001). An absolute rule approach. In Kuhse H and Singer P (ed.) *A companion to bioethics*. Blackwell Publishers, Oxford, 72–79.

Häyry M (2007). Utilitarianism and bioethics. In Ashcroft RE, Dawson A, Draper H and McMillan JR (ed.) *Principles of health care ethics* (2nd edn). John Wiley and Sons, Chichester, 57–64.

Hare R (2001). A utilitarian approach. In Kuhse H and Singer P (ed.) *A companion to bioethics*. Blackwell Publishers, Oxford, 80–85.

McNaughton DA and Rawling JP (2007). Deontology. In Ashcroft RE, Dawson A, Draper H and McMillan JR (ed.) *Principles of health care ethics* (2nd edn). John Wiley and Sons, Chichester, 65–71.

O'Neill O (2007). Kantian ethics. In Ashcroft RE, Dawson A, Draper H and McMillan JR (ed.) *Principles of health care ethics* (2nd edn). John Wiley and Sons, Chichester, 73–77.

Oakley J (2001). A virtue ethics approach. In Kuhse H and Singer P. (ed.) *A companion to bioethics*. Blackwell Publishers, Oxford, 86–97.

Oakley J (2007). Virtue theory. In Ashcroft RE, Dawson A, Draper H and McMillan JR (ed.) *Principles of health care ethics* (2nd edn). John Wiley and Sons, Chichester, 87–91.

Further reading

Doyal L (1999). Ethico-legal dilemmas within general practice, moral indeterminacy and abstract morality. In Dowrick C and Frith L (ed.) *General practice and ethics, uncertainty and responsibility*. Routledge, London.

Downie RS and Calman KC (1994). *Healthy respect: ethics in health care* (2nd edn). Oxford University Press, Oxford.

Chapter 3

Trust and the doctor–patient relationship

Introduction

Case 3.1

Soon after Dr Amy Walker's arrival at the St Andrew's practice in Dunedin, the receptionist asks if she could see an extra, a young child with a fever. Dr Walker agrees, and Mrs Barnes brings in her 2-year-old son Trevor, saying that he has been very flat with a fever since last night. On examination, Trevor is drowsy and febrile, with marked neck stiffness and photophobia. Dr Walker makes a diagnosis of meningitis and arranges for urgent transfer to Dunedin Hospital, giving a dose of antibiotics as recommended by the paediatric registrar on duty. At lunchtime, she tells Dr Mackenzie (the long-standing principal in the practice) of Trevor's illness, later confirmed by the hospital as bacterial meningitis. He and the practice nurse who is in the room fall inexplicably silent, until finally Dr Mackenzie explains: Mrs Barnes is regarded as a difficult patient/mother by the practice, frequently requesting urgent appointments and home visits for apparently trivial illnesses in her children. If the receptionist had rung Dr Mackenzie, he would not have seen Trevor urgently. Thinking about the possible consequences of a delay in treatment is a sobering experience for Dr Mackenzie.

In this chapter we examine the doctor–patient relationship in general practice. What kinds of values are important in this relationship, and in what ways can the relationship come to grief? We take trust to be central to the doctor–patient relationship; accordingly the first part of the chapter explores trust, looking at moral reasons for patients to trust doctors and doctors to trust patients. In the second part of the chapter, we look at issues that can arise when there are problems in the relationship. The material in this chapter is closely linked the contents of other chapters; there are specific cross-references to help you make these connections.

What is the doctor–patient relationship?

The meeting between patient and GP is at the centre of healthcare in general practice (McWhinney 1997). The consultation is the medium through which people access their GPs and through which GPs provide clinical care. Within the consultation, the nature and quality of the healthcare provided is largely dependent upon the nature and quality of the interaction. In most consultations, both accurate diagnosis and effective treatment rely upon the quality of the relationship between the doctor and patient (Kaba and Sookiakumaran 2007). The term 'doctor–patient relationship' refers to this specific interaction, which may be characterized in various ethical, medical and technical ways. The term also encompasses the important but hard to define bond that develops between patients and doctors over time, acting as the basis for specific interactions and allowing relative strangers to feel at ease in unusually intimate situations (Christie and Hoffmaster 1986; Kaba and Sookiakumaran 2007). Why is the relationship between doctor and patient so important, and why has it become one of the defining features of general practice?

It may be helpful if we think of the relationship as the substrate or foundation upon which care occurs. In a flourishing relationship, this foundation is strengthened over time and reinforced by positive interactions. This strong base then becomes capable of supporting major events, such as providing care through serious illnesses or ongoing support for chronic ill health. These are instrumental benefits of the doctor–patient relationship: with a well-functioning relationship, it is easier for the GP to provide better healthcare and outcomes may be improved. A lot of general practice research attempts to measure and define various aspects of the GP–patient relationship and relate these to outcomes such as patient satisfaction, compliance with treatment, patient recall of information and resolution of symptoms (Howie *et al.* 1999; Little *et al.* 2001; Flocke *et al.* 2002).

Trying to define the instrumental benefits of the relationship may distract our attention away from another important issue–the intrinsic value of the relationship. By intrinsic value, we mean that the relationship is of value in itself, over and above any measurable improvements in health outcomes or greater patient satisfaction. Of course, there is a lot more to say here; not all relationships are rosy and, like any other relationship, the one between a GP and a patient may be harmful or destructive. Our basic premise is that particular kinds of relationships are of value, and it is part of the task of ethics to work out just what is valuable in a 'good' GP–patient relationship.

The importance of the relationship to general practice

In Chapter 1 we briefly discussed the central role of the GP–patient relationship and reasons why it is considered so important. One of the main reasons for the centrality of the relationship is the ongoing commitment to individual persons, rather than to diseases or techniques, along with the holistic approach that this entails. Holistic care requires that GPs know their patients in a more thorough and robust way than for some other kinds of medical care. Finding out and using this information is part of a good relationship.

The continuing and open-ended nature of general practice provides the scope for relationships to evolve, in response to the changing needs and demands of both parties. GPs have to respond to any and all problems that patients present. This job becomes easier if GPs can draw upon their store of personal information about patients. In a good relationship there are established patterns of communication or behaviour, and each person knows more or less what to expect from the other. Drawing upon the capital of the relationship can help GPs to asses the urgency of symptoms: the onset of pain in a patient known for her stoicism and infrequent attendances will be taken far more seriously than an apparently similar pain in a patient with a different pattern of physical symptoms and level of anxiety about health.

Finally, much of general practice is concerned with problems that do not sort into neat pathophysiological conditions. Often the diagnosis is uncertain or the problem relates to psycho-social issues, or there is no 'medical' solution. In these cases, the GP herself is a therapeutic agent, and how well or ill the patient feels will depend upon the GP's skill at building the relationship. In cases where there may not be any specific medical action to take, the nature of the interaction and the relationship in which this is grounded assume relatively greater importance.

Of course, some of these features may be shared with other kinds of medical care, such as paediatrics or some branches of internal medicine, but no other speciality has embraced the doctor–patient relationship as a defining feature in the way of general practice.

Ethical interest in the doctor–patient relationship has focused upon defining particular features, in terms of rights and responsibilities, the character of the interaction, power issues and decision-making. There are many different ways to classify the relationship, but commonly this is done along a spectrum from consumerist to paternalistic (see Box 3.1).

These two extremes of the doctor–patient relationship are a useful way of drawing our attention to important ethical values in the relationship, such as acting for the patient's good, and respecting patients' autonomy. Beneficence and

Box 3.1 Consumerism and paternalism: the ethical extremes of the doctor–patient relationship

Consumerist

Consumerist relationships take the patient to be a client or consumer, and the doctor to be a technical adviser. Patients/consumers are in charge of their own health and have the right to as much information as they need to make their own decisions about healthcare. The doctor's role is to provide the best possible information to the patient so that the patient can decide what treatment they desire. The doctor may have a further role in helping the patient to implement their decision. Consumerist relationships are based upon the ethical value of respect for patient autonomy. The emphasis is upon patients making their own choices about what happens to them in terms of their healthcare.

Paternalistic

Paternalistic relationships are the opposite extreme. This model takes the patient to be vulnerable or helpless, in need of medical care and unable to make decisions. The doctor is seen as the all-powerful expert who knows what is best for the patient. It is the doctor's role to make decisions on behalf of the patient, who is a passive recipient of care. Paternalistic relationships are based upon the ethical value of beneficence or acting for the good of the patient. The emphasis is upon the duty of doctors to act in their patients' best interests.

respect for patient autonomy are important ethical values, but on their own they do not exhaust the range of values that may occur in the relationship. (For further discussion of beneficence and patient autonomy, see Chapters 6 and 8.) Empirical research with patients and doctors offers some interesting and contradictory insights into the kinds of relationships that patients prefer. In one study, between 65 and 78% of patients preferred a shared decision-making role, 20 to 34% preferred a passive role and only 1% preferred an autonomous role (Deber *et al.* 2007). Murray *et al.* (2007) had similar findings in relation to shared decision-making, which was preferred by 62% of respondents in their study; but they found that 28% of patients preferred a more consumerist model, with 9% preferring paternalism. However, Flynn *et al.* (2006) found a much higher rate of 57% of respondents who wanted to retain personal control over important medical decisions, with 39% in their study who preferred their physician to make important medical decisions.

It seems there is no single approach preferred by patients, nor is it clear that patient preferences are stable over time in this regard.

Shared decision-making is a half way position between consumerism and paternalism. Definitions of this vary but, at the least, it involves providing patients with information and encouraging their participation in the process of making decision about their care. The ethical benefits of shared decision-making are that it shows respect for patients by providing information, seeking understanding and promoting autonomy, whilst also demonstrating care and a commitment to the patient's wellbeing. There are also practical benefits, such as increased patient knowledge, greater compliance with treatment and better outcomes (Fraenkel and McGraw 2007). Shared decision-making in general practice has been described as idealistic, impractical and impossible (Elwyn 2006). Whilst it may not be possible to achieve this ideal in every consultation, there are some prerequisites (see Box 3.2) that are necessary for shared decision-making and through this, realization of the ethical goals of respect, being trustworthy and supporting patient autonomy.

Box 3.2 Prerequisites for patients to participate in shared decision-making

1. Adequate patient knowledge.
2. Explicit encouragement of patient participation by physicians.
3. Appreciation of the patient's right to play an active role in decision-making.
4. Awareness of choice.
5. Time (Fraenkel and McGraw 2007).

The importance of trust

We believe that trust is a central and crucial ethical value in the GP–patient relationship as, without trust, we cannot seek or provide healthcare. Trust operates in both directions: it is usually taken for granted that patients should trust their doctors, although what this means exactly is not always clear. Whether doctors should trust patients is a question that is asked less often. Before looking at the ways that trust influences the relationship, we need to spend a little time analysing what we mean by trust.

Trust is a way of dealing with uncertainty, a way of approaching relationships so that we can manage the risks of interactions with others. When we call someone trustworthy, we are usually commending them in some way. When we invite someone to trust us, we are making a statement about our motives, and our honesty and reliability. Trust involves being optimistic about the person trusted in two main ways:

1. Is the person competent to do what we trust them to do?
2. Does the person bear goodwill towards us, so that they will respect our trust and do what we are expecting them to do? (Jones 1996).

There is an inevitable element of risk in trusting another person, which creates vulnerability (Stirrat and Gill 2005). When we trust another person, we usually grant them quite a lot of discretionary powers, which of course may be used to help or harm the person trusting (Baier 1986). If we trust the neighbour to look after our house when we are on holiday, giving him the key allows him equally the power to harm us by stealing things or to help us by feeding the cat.

If we stop to think about it, consciously trusting another person involves examining our beliefs about that person, and making a judgement about the reasons we have for those beliefs (Holton 1994). But often we trust or distrust without really thinking, so that our trust or distrust may reflect our prejudices rather than a calm and cool evaluation of specific reasons to trust. Trusting can be a risky business (the neighbour may steal our heirlooms), but trust is a fundamental ingredient in relationships ranging from the politely co-operative through to intimate partnerships. One important feature of trust is the way that we feel if we are let down. If we really trusted the neighbour, we will feel very betrayed if they have stolen our possessions. This is in contrast to the annoyance or disappointment we might feel if we are merely relying on someone. For example, although we rely on the plumber to fix our tap, we do not usually trust him to come on time. When he is late, we might be annoyed but we do not feel betrayed. Trust leads to 'a readiness to feel betrayal should it be disappointed' (Holton 1994, p.67).

Trust in the doctor–patient relationship

What kinds of trust might occur in the relationship between GPs and their patients? We usually speak of patients trusting their doctors, and this can cover a number of areas. Patients' trust may relate to the competence or the goodwill or both of the GP. If we asked a patient about trusting their GP, she might say something like:

I trust him to work out what is wrong, and to know what to advise.

I trust that he is up to date with medical information and that, if he doesn't know what is wrong, he will refer me to someone else who does.

I trust that he will behave professionally and not betray confidential material or try to take advantage of my situation.

I trust that, when he recommends a treatment, it is because he believes this is the best treatment for me, and not because he is needs more patients for a drug trial.

I trust that he will provide medical care even if there is no cure for my illness.

The list could continue for longer, but even this brief start makes us realize the almost endless content of the trust that a patient might have in their GP.

Trust in one area need not extend to trust in other areas. A patient may trust the goodwill of their GP in terms of confidentiality, affability, honesty and the like, but may not trust their competence in some clinical areas. The practice nurse, for example, may be a much quicker and gentler syringer of ears than the GP. Conversely, a GP may be trusted to be competent with straightforward clinical problems such as hypertension or arthritis, but not with sensitive personal information about depression or abuse. From the GP's perspective, it might not always be obvious what it is that the GP is being trusted to do, so that trust may be unwittingly betrayed.

Case 3.2

Ms Marion Sims goes to see her GP, Dr Chu, because she has had recurrent headaches. Dr Chu takes a history and examines Ms Sims, and comes to a provisional diagnosis of tension headaches exacerbated by a recent changes of job. Ms Sims leaves the consultation dissatisfied. Her sister also had headaches and was referred for a CT scan of her head, and Ms Sims thinks she also should have a scan. She does not trust Dr Chu's diagnosis because she thinks he is just trying to save money by not referring her.

Dr Chu is unaware of Ms Sim's reasoning, and does not realize that she does not trust his diagnosis. If Dr Chu is competent in formulating his diagnosis, then this distrust is probably unwarranted, but it will be hard for him to regain trust unless he finds out exactly what Ms Sims expects, and explains to her why her case is not the same as her sister's.

Communication can have a significant impact upon trust. A study from the USA investigating racial differences in trust found that the communication of physicians with their patients varied according to race, affecting trust. Prior to visiting the doctor, both black and white patients had similar levels of trust in physicians. Following the consultations, black patients reported lower levels of trust, related to perceptions about less supportive and less informative communication (Gordon *et al.* 2006). Given the recognized importance of trust for patients in relation to their willingness to seek care, to disclose symptoms, to cooperate with treatment, to participate in research and to continue treatment with a particular doctor, communication that builds trust is crucial (Hall *et al.* 2001).

Does the reverse hold true, and should GPs trust patients? The issue of doctors trusting patients is less well-recognized, but we can identify at least three areas in which doctors should trust patients:

1. *Motive*: this is to do with trusting that patients are genuinely seeking medical care and share the aims of diagnosing and managing a health problem. A GP might distrust a patient's motives if she thinks the patient is acting for some other reason, such as malice, or to obtain access to drugs of dependence, or sick certification.

2. *Testimony*: this is to do with trusting that patients are telling the truth without too many exaggerations or omissions; for example, that the pain was as severe as reported and not an exaggeration to obtain more time off work or stronger pain killers.

3. *Competence*: this is to do with trusting that patients are competent, both in the general sense of understanding information and in the practical sense of being able to cooperate with management (Rogers 2002).

Being trusted feels good: patients who are accepted at face value and whose histories are believed, feel validated by this. Trust provides a moral boost, together with reassurance that they are right to have consulted the doctor. In contrast, seeing a doctor who does not believe the history or who thinks the patient is malingering is a very difficult experience. In Case 3.1, at the start of this chapter, Dr Walker's colleague no longer trusted Mrs Barnes to know when to call for a doctor, and his lack of trust in her testimony and competence might have led to tragic consequences. Dr Walker had no reason to doubt Mrs Barnes' request for an urgent appointment, and her basic trust in patients knowing when they need medical care may have saved Trevor's life.

The benefits of trust

There are important ethical reasons why trust is important in the doctor–patient relationship. A willingness to trust is ethically valuable because trusting another person involves treating that person as a moral agent. Trusting implies that the person trusted is capable of taking responsibility for their decisions (Horsburgh 1960). A GP who trusts her patient has taken the necessary ethical step of recognizing the patient as a person, rather than seeing her as a passive recipient of care. This recognition of the individuality and capacities of the patient is a necessary part of respect for autonomy. It is also a central part of the holistic philosophy of general practice, and important in developing the GP–patient relationship (May and Mead 1999). Withholding trust denies patients the opportunity to act as responsible moral agents in relation to their own healthcare decisions.

Trust may be therapeutic, in the sense that trusting a person may increase their trustworthiness, by positively influencing the trusted person's behaviour. In this sense, trust is a kind of moral support, allowing the person who is trusted the chance to live up to expectations. This kind of trust may occur, for example, in a relationship between a GP and a person with a dependence disorder. Sometimes extending trust in this situation can provide the moral encouragement that the patient needs to make therapeutic progress. In this situation trust is both a practical and an ethical approach to influencing behaviour constructively. Trust in this situation can be risky, as the other person may not be able to live up to those expectations. But just as people may live up to expectations, they may also live down to them. Never trusting a person prevents that person from ever showing that they have become trustworthy.

Trust offers a way of altering the power imbalance in the doctor–patient relationship. In most situations, it is the patient who lacks authority, recognized expertise and medical agency. They are also the one who is ill and they are often at a socio-economic disadvantage. By offering trust, the doctor can shift this balance of power. This can occur in a number of ways. Listening to patients and accepting their accounts of ill health demonstrates trust in their testimony; this is particularly important if the patient has confusing or unusual symptoms that may otherwise be dismissed. Trusting patients' motives is important, as the degree of trust is likely to influence the GP's response to the patient. Imagine a patient with a work-related back injury. If she is well-known to the GP and trusted, her care will reflect this and her GP will provide moral as well as medical support in her rehabilitation. However, an unknown patient may not be trusted in this way, losing both the moral and medical support. Similarly, patients who are trusted to be competent are given greater control over their treatment; for example, to manage their own insulin requirements. This is important in terms of creating the opportunities for patients to exercise autonomy and to regain some sense of individual control, which may have been compromised by being ill. On the other hand, if patients are distrusted by their GPs, the burden of that distrust is added to the original health problem, creating a reactive cycle of hostility and inhibiting good communication and clinical care.

As well as these ethical reasons, there are a number of obvious practical benefits if there are high levels of trust in the GP–patient relationship. Communication is easier, with less need to challenge or check up on statements, and less anxiety about what can be said, for both doctor and patient. With trust, it is easier to define the goals of the consultation. In trusting relationships, patients are able to accept the frequent uncertainty that accompanies diagnoses (or lack of diagnoses) in general practice. The presence of trust gives the GP some discretionary latitude, which is an advantage in an area as unpredictable as medicine. It is not always, or even often, possible to describe all of the potential outcomes or arrange plans to cover these contingencies, but in the presence of trust, both the GP and the patient can be sure that the other will exercise appropriate discretion. Thus a patient not specifically warned about a rare side-effect can be trusted to notify the GP should this occur, in turn trusting that he will welcome her observation and respond appropriately.

A relationship characterized by trust provides the flexibility to meet the variable demands of changes over time and in health status experienced by patients. Part of the problem with consumerist or paternalistic models of the doctor–patient relationship is that both parties are locked into a certain way of relating, that may not suit changing circumstances.

Case 3.3

Mr Lincoln is a healthy 42-year-old who sees his GP, Dr Day, infrequently, usually to discuss his preventive care options for the extensive travelling that he does. His relationship with Dr Day, developed over a number of years, follows a consumerist pattern: he asks for the medical information and goes away to decide which precautions to take, taking into account other factors such as the kinds of places that he usually stays in and his budget. If he decides to have a vaccination or take malaria prophylaxis, he rings the surgery and asks for a prescription to be arranged. This relationship suits Mr Lincoln as he likes to be well-informed and make his own decisions.

However, Mr Lincoln becomes very unwell, with weakness, fatigue, weight loss and night sweats. When Dr Day tells him of the tests that are necessary to reach a diagnosis, Mr Lincoln hears only the words 'possible malignancy' and becomes very frightened. He doesn't want to go away and do his own research and make his own decision. He wants Dr Day to be in control, trusting him to make the appropriate choices about investigations. Later, after the acute phase of the illness, he regains his confidence and takes more control over his treatment.

If Dr Day had insisted on following the usual pattern of their relationship, we would consider him quite unfeeling and unresponsive to Mr Lincoln's drastic change in circumstances. Patients and GPs in strictly consumerist relationship would have trouble dealing with new situations if they lacked the trust to relate in new ways. However, Mr Lincoln knew Dr Day well enough to trust him in this crisis and, on the basis of this trust, to follow whatever advice he gave. Patients who are in relationships based upon trust are able to share the decision-making responsibility, trusting the GP to know and act in their interests.

Similarly, a relationship locked into a paternalistic pattern may have difficulty accommodating a patient's growing expertise as, for example, she becomes used to handling her disease and develops her own management strategies. When circumstances change, previously satisfactory patterns of relating may no longer be suitable. The presence of trust creates a climate in which changes in the relationship can occur more easily than if trust is absent, easing the transition into new ways of relating. Across the spectrum of relationships, trust acts as a safety net.

Trust, paternalism and consumerist relationships

One way of thinking about the role of trust in doctor–patient relationships is to identify what it is that makes some relationships ethically unacceptable. Paternalistic relationships are problematic when the doctor assumes control over the relationship, irrespective of the wishes of the patient. We can think of this as an imbalance of trust: the doctor is demanding trust from the patient, trust in the medical view about what is wrong and trust in the GP's competence at treating it. At the same time, the doctor is withholding any reciprocal trust in the patient's capacities and not respecting her competence for making decisions or managing her illness. On the other hand, we can imagine paternalistic relationships in which the patient willingly and justifiably trusts the doctor to act in her best interests, and the doctor proceeds because he knows that this is just what he is trusted to do. (See Chapter 6 for a full discussion of paternalism.)

Consumerist relationships seem to be an attempt to exclude trust. The doctor is not trusted for her opinions or to recommend options for the patient, and her obligation to provide information is seen as a contractual rather than moral obligation. In the absence of any trust, this is likely to lead to impersonal medical care. For consumerist relationships to work in a morally robust way, the patient has to be able to trust the information provided by the doctor, and the doctor has to trust the patient enough to provide the necessary information, and then trust them to make their own decision. Both consumerist and paternalistic relationships can be based upon trust, making them ethically acceptable.

Fostering patient trust

Doctors tend to assume that patients will trust them, and often this is the case. It is, however, possible to foster trust by being explicit about the grounds for trust. Fostering trust in the GP's competence involves both technical and moral elements. Taking care in explaining diagnostic and treatment options, the evidence for these where appropriate and the likely implications can demonstrate the trustworthiness of the GP's technical skills to the patient. Demonstrating moral competence includes being respectful of the autonomy of patients, recognizing their rights and facilitating meaningful participation in their healthcare.

Demonstrating goodwill may involve being explicit about the GP's commitment to the health and wellbeing of the patient, honouring any promises made to patients, being reliable and consistent over time, respecting patients' views and testimony, and maintaining the relationship on a professional level (McLeod 2004). Being explicit about fostering trust may feel initially awkward, but demonstrating trustworthiness, especially in situations where patients may have good reasons to withhold trust, is the key for building morally sound relationships.

Trusting wisely

Unfortunately, the presence of trust does not guarantee an ethical relationship. People make mistakes and trust when they should not, or withhold trust from others who are trustworthy. Trust and distrust colour the way we see the other person and, as in the case of Mrs Barnes and Trevor, can make it difficult to see past our habitual expectations. What are some ways to trust wisely?

First, we can look at the motives of the person who is being trusted, to see if there are any conflicts between their motives and the demands of trustworthiness. For example, if a GP is being paid generously by a pharmaceutical company to recruit patients into a drug trial, patients might question the trustworthiness of that GP if she encourages them to take part in the trial. Similarly, if a patient with opioid dependence is seeking treatment for an apparently painful condition, the GP may rightly question the trustworthiness of the patient's account. Patients, however, do not have reliable ways of finding information about GPs' potentially conflicting motives. This creates an imperative for GPs to be honest with about their motives, with their patients as well as themselves. We deal with conflicts of interest in greater detail in Chapter 12.

Next, we can examine our own reasons for thinking that the other person is or is not trustworthy. Prejudice and stereotyping can bias our views about the trustworthiness of others. This can work both ways in the GP–patient relationship.

Patients' assumptions about general practice may prevent them from trusting the GP's motives. The withholding of antibiotics for viral illnesses, or X-rays for low back pain, may be interpreted as cost-saving rather than good medical care. GPs may make assumptions about the honesty or competence of patients based on unreflective generalizations rather than consciously weighing the reasons for trusting or not trusting in each case.

Trusting someone who is untrustworthy usually means that one person is being deceptive, potentially exploiting the person who is trusting. These are unwelcome ethical harms in themselves, but it is also worth looking at the consequences of misplaced trust in the doctor–patient relationship. For GPs, if a patient has been deceptive, there is the risk that the doctor's time and efforts are wasted or misplaced; for example, through trying to find an organic cause for a fictitious complaint. There is also the risk that the patient will come to harm; for example, if a complaint of pain motivated by opiate dependence is taken on trust as 'genuine' pain, the patient is harmed through misdiagnosis and further access to opiates. Doctors often feel betrayed by dependent patients; this seems to reflect professional vulnerability, as not recognizing a dependent patient can be seen as a professional failing. These harms from trusting untrustworthy patients are borne by the GP. In other cases, however, the risks are borne by society rather than the individual doctor. For example, if a patient gains unjustified access to sickness benefits or compensation, it is the social welfare system rather than the doctor him or herself who has to pay the benefits.

For patients, the risks of trusting an untrustworthy doctor can be far more direct and personal. In extreme cases, misplaced trust can lead to death, either through incompetence or, very unusually, malice. Usually the consequences are not so drastic, but it is hard to measure the kind of harm that occurs when a doctor is untrustworthy due to incompetence or lack of goodwill. Patients cannot always judge competence, and doctors are often loathe to blow the whistle on their colleagues. This professional silence, as well as protecting untrustworthy doctors, may also foster a more general distrust of doctors.

Conclusion

In this chapter we have proposed a perhaps idealistic doctor–patient relationship based upon trust. Trust plays a crucial role, both moral and practical, in doctor–patient relationships. Relationships based on warranted trust may range from paternalistic to consumerist; in these cases it is the presence of reciprocal trust that makes the relationships morally acceptable. Trust is easy to withhold, but when patients are not trusted, this can hamper good medical care, as well as impose extra burdens upon patients. These observations about trust imply that there is an obligation for GPs to consciously, and demonstrably, be trustworthy, and to trust patients unless there are justifiable reasons for withholding trust.

Trusting patients will not necessarily transform all GP–patient relationships into rosy ones, but consciously thinking about trust can help to flesh out some of the moral responsibilities that both doctors and patients have towards each other, making it easier to consider other important ethical issues that occur in practice. In the next chapter we discuss what happens when things go wrong in the relationship.

References

Baier A (1986). Trust and antitrust. *Ethics* **96**, 231–260.

Christie R and Hoffmaster B (1986). *Ethical issues in family medicine.* New York, Oxford University Press.

Deber R, Kraetschmer N, Urowitz S and Sharpe N (2007). Do people want to be autonomous patients? Preferred roles in treatment decision-making in several patient populations. *Health Expectations* **10**(3), 248–258.

Elwyn G (2006). Idealistic, impractical, impossible? Shared decision-making in the real world. *British Journal of General Practice* **56**(527), 403–404.

Flocke SA, Miller WL and Crabtree BF (2002). Relationships between physician practice style, patient satisfaction, and attributes of primary care. *Journal of Family Practice* **51**, 835–840.

Flynn K, Smith M and Freese J (2006). When do older adults turn to the internet for health information? Findings from the Wisconsin Longitudinal Study. *Journal of General Internal Medicine* **21**(12), 1295–1301.

Fraenkel L and McGraw S (2007). What are the essential elements to enable patient participation in medical decision-making? *Journal of General Internal Medicine* **22**(5), 614–619.

Gordon HS, Street RL, Sharf BF, Kelly A and Souchek J (2006). Racial differences in trust and lung cancer patients' perceptions of physician communication. *Journal of Clinical Oncology* **24**, 904–909.

Hall MA, Dugan E, Zheng B and Mishra AK (2001). Trust in physicians and medical institutions, what is it, can it be measured, and does it matter? *The Milbank Quarterly* **79**, 613–619.

Holton R (1994). Deciding to trust, coming to believe. *Australasian Journal of Philosophy* **72**, 63–76.

Horsburgh H (1960). The ethics of trust. *The Philosophical Quarterly* **10**, 343–354.

Howie JG, Heaney DJ, Maxwell M, Walker JJ, Freeman GK and Rai H (1999). Quality at general practice consultations, cross sectional survey. *British Medical Journal* **319**, 738–743.

Jones K (1996). Trust as an Affective Attitude. *Ethics* **107**, 4–25.

Kaba R and Sooriakumaran (2007). The evolution of the doctor–patient relationship. *International Journal of Surgery* **5**, 57–65.

Little P, Everitt H, Williamson I, Warner G, Moore M, Gould C, Ferrier K and Payne S (2001). Observational study of effect of patient centredness and positive approach on outcomes of general practice consultations. *British Medical Journal* **323**, 908–911.

May C and Mead N (1999). Patient-centredness, a history. In Dowrick C and Frith L (ed.) *General practice and ethics, uncertainty and responsibility*. Routledge, London and New York, 91–106.

McLeod C (2004). Understanding trust. In Bayliss F, Downie J, Hoffmaster B and Sherwin S (ed.) *Healthcare ethics in Canada* (2nd edn). Thomson Nelson, Toronto, Canada, 186–191.

McWhinney I (1997). *A textbook of family medicine* (2nd edn). Oxford University Press, New York.

Murray E, Pollack L, White M, Lo, B (2007. Clinical decision-making, Patients' preferences and experiences. *Patient Education & Counseling*. **65**(2), 189–96.

Rogers WA (2002). Is there a moral duty to trust patients? *Journal of Medical Ethics* **28**, 77–80.

Stirrat, GM and Gill R (2005). Autonomy in medical ethics after O'Neill. *Journal of Medical Ethics* **31**, 127–130.

Chapter 4

Difficult relationships with patients

Introduction

A well-functioning doctor–patient relationship tends to drop out of sight, with straightforward communication, productive negotiations and apparently effortless decision-making. In reality, the situation can be much more difficult. Relationships may become challenging if there are tensions between intimacy and professionalism, if there are relationships that extend beyond the consultation or if unacceptable gifts are offered. Sexual attractions between doctors and patients raise ethical issues, as do relationships with patients who are very dependent or needy. In this chapter we explore some of the challenges when relationships with patients become difficult.

The balance between intimacy and professionalism

One of the most difficult areas concerns the limits and boundaries of the relationship between GP and patient. In the previous chapter we outlined an ideal relationship of mutual trust and respect, but is it realistic to expect this kind of relationship to remain strictly limited to the consulting room? How should caring and involved GPs reach the appropriate balance between intimacy and professionalism with their patients? These issues are explored in the following sections, but first we must discuss why boundaries are important. The term 'boundary' refers to the distinction between professional and personal identity. There is a need to make this distinction as the roles and responsibilities that attach to each of these identities differ. Boundaries exist to keep those on either side safe (Sarkar 2004). The professional identity of the doctor allows the patient to be safe within the consultation, despite any disclosures of private information or examination of intimate parts of the body. Likewise, the professional role allows doctors to engage in these acts without fear of prosecution. Maintaining boundaries is crucial for trustworthy and ethical healthcare. The most serious boundary violations involve sexual relationships with patients, but there are other ways in which the integrity of the relationship can be breached.

The doctor–patient relationship may reach beyond the consulting room in a number of ways. Patients may have relationships with their GP in other contexts, such as in community work or on committees. Sometimes even acknowledging patients outside the consultation can breach confidentiality, unless the greeting is initiated by the patient. It seems unreasonable to avoid any social interaction with people who are also patients, but at the same time the GP must try to distinguish between any social roles and their role as GP. This might require discussion with the other person, to clarify how best to balance professionalism within a developing friendship. Limiting discussion of health issues to the consultation is a common sense way of protecting the boundary, as well maintaining confidentiality. At times it can be hard to maintain the boundaries, especially when different relationships require different roles. A patient who is in a more casual role in one context may find the greater formality of the doctor–patient relationship difficult to adjust to, as may the GP involved. Problems in one relationship may spill over into other unrelated areas, leading to questions about when the doctor–patient relationship may be considered over, as in Case 4.1.

Case 4.1

Miss Little has a longstanding relationship with her GP, Dr John Buchan. Miss Little and Dr Buchan are members of the same Dunedin community arts committee, which meets frequently. Miss Little has a chronic illness, for which she also sees a complementary therapist. The therapist advises a course of prescribed medication, available only through a GP. Dr Buchan and his partner, Dr Mackenzie, have decided on a policy of not providing this treatment as it is not considered medically effective and is also very expensive. This refusal eventually leads to Miss Little changing to another practice.

However, Dr Buchan has ongoing contact with Miss Little through their community arts work. In this context, Miss Little is hostile and angry with Dr Buchan, and indicates to other members of the committee that she has been badly treated by the St Andrew's practice. This creates a problem for Dr Buchan. Should he continue to maintain the tenor of the doctor–patient relationship, even though Miss Little is no longer a patient, or should he respond as he would to any person he is finding difficult to work with on the committee?

There are some options open to Dr Buchan in this situation. Miss Little's medical information is confidential, so he cannot counter the charges with his own account of what has happened. Dr Buchan can attempt to discuss the issue with Miss Little and ask her to separate the issues related to her medical care from their current work on the committee. If this is not successful, he is no longer morally obliged to treat Miss Little with the consideration that he would give to a patient. Dr Buchan should be free to interact with Miss Little simply as a difficult committee member. However, it would be prudent for him to discuss the issue with a peer or a representative of a medical regulatory body, to protect himself against a formal complaint from Miss Little.

Information disclosed within the GP–patient relationship can have an impact upon the GP's personal life. For example, within the consultation a GP may become aware that a female patient is involved in an extra-marital affair. If this patient is also a close friend of the GP's partner, it can be hard for the GP to separate the professional from the personal. How should he react to the patient/friend of his wife in social situations, and should he withhold the information if his wife voices suspicion about her friend's marriage? The GP's obligation to the patient includes confidentiality, but he may consider asking her to change GPs if he feels that her ongoing care is causing tensions within his own intimate relationships. (See Chapter 5 for a full discussion of confidentiality.)

Within the consultation, GPs hold much more personal knowledge about their patients than the other way around. Sharing some personal information with patients can be a way of strengthening the relationship and building trust, but this can also be the beginning of the 'slippery slope' towards inappropriate boundary violations (Sarkar 2004). Some patients are the sorts of people that we are usually friends with, so that it seems natural to tell them something about personal events, but it is necessary to be aware of one's own emotions and motives in order to understand why these disclosures are being made at this time, with this patient.

Issues of friendship with patients are perhaps most significant in isolated settings, where it may be inevitable that the GP's friends will also be his or her patients. It may not be feasible or desirable to avoid treating one's friends in this situation, nor to avoid friendships with people who are also patients. Boundaries may blur between the role of friend and that of doctor but it is usually possible to separate the roles within the relationship; for example, by refusing to be drawn into medical matters except in a formal consultation, and avoiding discussion of friendship-related matters during consultations. These are artificial barriers to some extent, but they are important to preserve the integrity of both the medical relationship and the friendship.

Gifts from patients

Most GPs will experience gift giving by patients, perhaps after a period of intense care or an event such as a birth or death, or in recognition of seasonal festivities.

Gift giving may be motivated by various factors ranging from cultural traditions or the natural expression of goodwill, through to attempts to secure special treatment or to develop a more intimate relationship with the GP. What are the ethical issues raised by receiving such gifts? Perhaps the most important is that of justice and equity (Spence 2005). Only some patients can afford to give gifts and there is a danger that receiving gifts will influence the doctor to act more favourably towards those patients compared with others who do not bring gifts. Such favouritism might be expressed through longer or more frequent consultations or priority treatment, all of which may be unjust to other patients. Accepting gifts may make the GP feel indebted to the patient in ways that interfere with good medical care; for example, clouding diagnostic judgement or being less persistent with some aspects of history taking. Finally, accepting gifts may create a dangerous intimacy within the relationship, leading to the possibility of more serious boundary violations.

Many patients offer small gifts to their GPs, such as home-made jam or articles of clothing for the GP's newly arrived baby. Refusing these gifts can seem heartless and unnecessary, and may risk offending the patient, causing damage to the doctor–patient relationship. Problems may arise, however, when the gifts are inappropriately generous or seem to be given for an ulterior motive. Some gifts may not be directly related to medical care but may be attempts to gain an advantage in business dealings with the practice. Most professional bodies, such as the General Medical Council, offer advice on receiving gifts when there is a possible conflict of interest, stating that doctors should not put themselves in a position in which their judgement about a patient's care could be questioned with regard to any party from whom they have received gifts (General Medical Council 2006a). Given that doctors have an ethical duty to make the care of the patient their first concern, there is no theoretical advantage in giving a gift to secure better care! Advice from the British Medical Association indicates that GPs should keep a register of gifts with a value of over £100 (British Medical Association 2007). However, it is not clear that the influence of gifts is related to their monetary value. One common rule-of-thumb is to refuse any gift unless you would be willing for information about that gift to be made public. Many practices avoid the potential difficulties associated with gifts from patients by having a practice policy covering issues such as acceptable limits of gifts and the distribution of gifts either to charitable institutions (local hospital or old people's home) or to practice staff (Champ et al. 1995). Any policy on gifts should be publicized to patients. This kind of approach is preferable to an opportunistic approach in which only unwanted gifts are passed on.

Is it always unethical to accept gifts? Perhaps the most difficult situation arises when a patient wills a significant gift to their GP. An elderly person with no close relatives might prefer to leave particular items, such as books, to a well-known and liked GP rather than to a distant relative or to a charity. Accepting a gift in this circumstance will not affect the GP's judgement with regard to the patient, as the patient is dead. Ethically speaking, accepting the gift might be a way of respecting and honouring that patient's memory. Decisions about accepting gifts willed by patients need to be made by the individual involved, bearing in mind possible accusations of unprofessionalism or trial by media. What might actually be an ethical response in terms of accepting the books may be distorted or misrepresented to the GP's detriment. The issue of gifts from the pharmaceutical industry is covered in Chapter 12.

Sexual boundary violations

Almost any relationship offers opportunities for sexual involvement and the doctor–patient relationship is no exception. Although accurate figures are difficult to come by, the literature indicates that between 3 and 10% of doctors admit to a sexual relationship with patients (Galletly 2004). This is likely to be an underestimate, as patients who have been sexually exploited may not wish to pursue a complaint for reasons including shame, fear of not being believed, lack of resources necessary for participation in a formal investigation and lack of evidence. Sexual boundary violations are amongst the most serious professional offences and are severely punished both by the professional regulatory bodies and the courts.

What are the ethical considerations here? As discussed above, boundaries keep those on either side safe and help to maintain the appropriate roles of both patient and doctor. Sexual boundary violations lead to a number of significant harms. For the patient, sexual boundary violations can be extremely destructive. The abuse of a position of trust for sexual gratification triggers responses similar to those following incest. These include shame, guilt, rage, depression, self-harm and suicidality, substance misuse, sexual dysfunction, identity confusion, paranoia and break-up of relationships (Galletly 2004; Sarkar 2004). Subsequent distrust may preclude future therapeutic relationships, and this may be compounded by a lack of handover following an abrupt termination of the sexual relationship with the treating practitioner. In ethical terms, sexual boundary violations are a betrayal of trust, contravening the duties to act in the patient's best interests and to do no harm.

The harms for doctors are likewise significant. These include trauma and shame associated with investigation of the offences, loss of medical registration and loss of income, damage to family relationships and public humiliation.

Does this mean that it can never be ethical to have a sexual relationship with a person who is also a patient? Most regulatory bodies have zero tolerance towards sexual relationships with current patients (see, for example: General Medical Council 2006b; Medical Council of New Zealand 2006), for the reasons outlined above. If there is mutual attraction with a current patient, the main ethical consideration must be the interests of the patient and avoiding any situation that exploits the patient or compromises their care. Ideally, if there is a growing attraction between GP and patient, this should be acknowledged and the patient transferred to the care of another doctor, before the relationship develops any further. However, it would be very difficult to ensure that the relationship was not influenced by the dynamics and power imbalances of the consultation, which would undermine the validity of any consent given by the patient for sexual activity, even if a lengthy waiting period was observed.

The issue of relationships with former patients is ethically less clear, although these also carry risks of harm and are unethical if the doctor uses any power imbalance, knowledge or influence that derived from the previous professional relationship to pursue the patient (Medical Council of New Zealand 2006). Relationships with former patients may be acceptable depending upon the nature of the initial therapeutic interactions, the length of the practitioner–patient relationship and so forth; some commentators, however, argue strongly that these relationships are rarely ethically permissible due to the persistence of transference (Hall 2001).

Is it always an abuse of medical power if a GP first meets a person as a patient, and then pursues the relationship outside the context of medical care? For example, in isolated communities, it may be impossible to meet someone who is not, and has never been, a patient. It is impossible to give an answer that covers all potential situations, but in general GPs should be extremely wary of attractions that commence within the doctor–patient relationship. In addition, it would be prudent to discuss the issue with a colleague and the relevant medical regulatory body.

Situations of one-sided attraction require sensitive handling.

Case 4.2

Dr Mira Singh has not been in Wilford long before she realizes that one of her patients, Brett Fielding, has become infatuated with her. Mira and Brett meet socially through a shared interest in local bushland preservation, and on these occasions Brett makes comments about Mira's attractiveness. Dr Singh gains real pleasure from her bush care activities, so she does not want to discontinue her involvement. At the same time, she does not want to do anything to encourage Mr Fielding or to foster intimacy. One day, Mr Fielding consults with a number of problems, one of which requires rectal examination.

In this situation, there are a number of considerations. The first is to provide the patient with the care he needs, and the second is to respect Dr Singh's right to practise without feeling forced into uncomfortable personal situations. Referring the patient to her partner Dr Day for his rectal examination is one way of avoiding unwanted physical intimacy, while continuing herself with less intimate care. This may be possible without directly raising the subject of the patient's feelings for Dr Singh. In general, early discussions with colleagues or partners reduce the burden upon the GP and provide support in finding an acceptable solution. What if the situation is reversed, so that it is the GP who is attracted to the patient who remains unaware of the attraction or does not welcome it? Proceeding with intimate examinations in this context betrays the patient's trust that the interaction is solely to meet their medical needs. Doctors must be aware of their feelings and act swiftly to avoid situations in which boundary violations may occur.

Box 4.1 Danger signs for sexual boundary violations

Seeing patients at unusual times or in special circumstances, especially when other staff are not present.

Asking patient to book the last appointment of the day.

Increasing length of consultations.

Increasing informality in the consultation, including use of first names.

Contacts outside the consultation, e.g. invitations for social interactions.

Revealing intimate details and personal information to the patient, especially of a sexual nature.

Touching or hugging patient.

Most discussions of sex and the doctor–patient relationship focus upon the vulnerability and/or exploitation of patients. However, there are situations in which GPs may become victims of sexual harassment or stalking. In a Canadian survey of female GPs, well over two-thirds of the respondents reported some kind of harassment, ranging from suggestive looks and sexual remarks through to rape (Schneider and Phillips 1997). As the authors discuss, there is a wide variety of forms sexual harassment of female GPs, some of which are specific to the role of being a general practitioner. They note the complex power relations in this situation: the doctor has the power and authority of her position as a medical practitioner, but patients are capable of wielding significant power when invoking their (male) gender roles. At the same time, there are limited formal avenues for GPs to respond to harassing behaviours of patients.

General practice can create very vulnerable situations in which GPs are alone with patients, sometimes in the patient's home. A general duty of care and the requirements of justice suggest that GPs should see any patient needing healthcare. However, sexual harassment or stalking by patients is a betrayal of the medical relationship. GPs of both sexes are entitled to take any necessary actions to be safe in their work. These include not disclosing any personal information to patients, maintaining clear professional boundaries, not working alone in the practice, documentation and reporting of any offences, referring the patient to another practitioner for ongoing care, and seeking support from colleagues and other parties, such as medical defence organizations (Pathe *et al.* 2002).

Needy or dependent patients

Many GPs experience difficulties in their relationships with patients who have needs that are hard to meet in the medical context. These might be patients with medically unexplained symptoms, or with minor mental illnesses or dependence disorders. Patients with these problems often leave the GP feeling helpless and inadequate, as whatever they suggest does not seem to alleviate the patient's problems. What is the ethical response of the GP in this situation? Issues of trust, respect for patient autonomy and acting in the patient's best interests can be hard to sort out. What does a patient with unexplained symptoms trust the GP to do, and in what ways should the GP trust the patient? A basic ethical requirement here is to trust that the patient is in distress and is making a genuine request for help. This can be difficult in the face of unacknowledged psychological illness, or denial about dependence. In the early stages of the relationship it may not be possible to trust the patient's testimony or competence. To build a therapeutic relationship however, the GP must trust that, at some level, the request for help is genuine. Once the GP has accepted that the patient wants help with a problem, she can then consider other ethical aspects, such as the potential to benefit or harm the patient, and how the patient's autonomy can be respected.

Case 4.3

Julian Servante is a 35-year-old male patient who is well known to Dr Carter. He has multiple problems including headaches, irritable bowel syndrome, joint pains and tiredness. His symptoms increase at times of stress, such as moving house and increased pressure at work. In the past, Dr Carter has performed many investigations including blood tests, abdominal X-rays and a CT scan of the head. All investigations have been normal but, despite this, Mr Servante remains anxious and feeling unwell and makes frequent requests for referrals, especially to a neurologist and to a gastroenterologist.

We can consider Dr Carter's possible actions in terms of the patient's needs and any potential harms and benefits. There seems little doubt that patients with medically unexplained symptoms are in distress with high rates of medical and physical dysfunction (Smith *et al.* 2003), and are in need of care. The ethical issue is how to care for such patients in ways that avoid harm and provide some relief to the patient. Investigations can exclude serious or urgent pathology and may alleviate some of the patient's anxiety. On the other hand, some investigations are potentially harmful, such as endoscopy or multiple X-rays, and all run the risk of false-positive or negative results, with subsequent iatrogenic consequences.

There is a developing literature on the management of patients with medically unexplained symptoms, who are estimated to comprise up to 30% of all general practice patients (Rosendal and Olesen 2005), and a developing consensus on the importance of communication in the management of these patients (Smith *et al.* 2003). Building trust through open and honest communication ensures that the patient receives the therapeutic benefits of an ongoing doctor–patient relationship. This does not mean that the GP must offer an open-ended response; part of the therapeutic response will almost certainly require setting limits. What is ethically required are respectful and honest responses about what the GP can do, acknowledging the limits of medical approaches but offering ongoing care despite the limitations. Recognizing the value of building a relationship may alleviate some of the pressure that GPs feel to 'do something', sparing both patients and the public purse the cost of unfruitful investigations and referrals.

Patients and their relatives

Providing care to families as well as individuals can lead to challenges, especially where there is a conflict between the interests of the patients concerned. Imagine a woman caring for her 84-year-old mother who is mildly demented and tends to wander at night. The daughter requests a sedative, both to keep her mother safe in bed at night and also to allow her to have peaceful nights. There are several considerations that are important with this kind of request. First, the GP has to determine the nature and extent of the problem. This can be difficult if the history is only available from the carer and it is possible that she is exaggerating in order to make sure her request is successful. The GP has to make an assessment about the trustworthiness of the carer, based on her previous knowledge of both her and her mother. It is also important to work out who the patient is in this context–is it the mother, who may be in danger from wandering, or the daughter, who is not getting enough sleep? A home visit may be necessary to assess the kinds of dangers that are present in the home. The request may be a cry for help from the carer, which she hopes will trigger a move towards residential care for her mother. Factors of this kind all feed into an ethical response and, as with other situations, there may be no ideal solution. Some kind of weighing up of the harms of sedatives versus the benefits of avoiding a nocturnal accident will be part of the decision, as will an assessment of the mother's understanding of the situation and willingness to take sleeping tablets.

Collusive relationships

As we have discussed above, the doctor–patient relationship can be an important therapeutic tool, providing the foundation for healthcare. However, sometimes the relationship can seem take on a life of its own, and both GP and patient may become locked into a relationship that meets some needs, but not perhaps the needs of healthcare. Collusion can develop when the GP acts from a desire to please the patient or preserve the relationship at any cost, rather than acting for the medical good of the patient. Collusion may initially seem harmless, such as agreeing with a patient's medically bizarre account of their symptoms. The situation becomes more difficult if patients request investigations or therapies that are not, according to current standards of evidence, medically effective and/or warranted in the circumstances. Giving in to these kind of requests may seem an attractive course of action, as pleasing people is far easier than refusing them, and there may be harm to the relationship if the refusal is seen as unwarranted by the patient. Collusion may also occur if the doctor is frightened of the patient, either physically or in terms of complaints or litigation. Balanced against these factors are the ethical requirements to act for the medical good of the patient and to be trustworthy rather than deceptive. Agreeing to provide medically unwarranted services is generally dishonest and undermines the growth of morally decent trust.

Conclusion

In this chapter we have discussed some of the challenges when relationships with patients become difficult. The difficulties may range from extremely serious boundary violations through to unwilling collusion with needy patients, and encompass balancing friendships with providing medical care. These kinds of difficulties are not the norm in practice, but can lead to devastating consequences at times. Part of the skill of general practice lies in being aware of the ways in which difficulties can arise, and acting to avoid them where possible.

References

British Medical Association, General Practitioners Committee (2007). *Accepting donations from patients*. Published by the British Medical Association.

Champ R, Haslam D and Lewis W (1995). A patient who keeps giving expensive gifts. *Practitioner* **239**, 695–698.

Galletly CA (2004). Crossing professional boundaries in medicine: the slippery slope to patient sexual exploitation. *Medical Journal of Australia* **181**, 380–383.

General Medical Council (2006a). *Good medical practice* (paragraphs 72c and 74). Available at http://www.gmc-uk.org/guidance/good_medical_practice/index.asp (accessed 19 August 2008).

General Medical Council (2006b). *Maintaining boundaries*. Available at http://www. gmc-uk.org/guidance/current/library/maintaining_boundaries.asp#4 (accessed 19 August 2008).

Hall KH (2001). Sexualization of the doctor–patient relationship: is it ever ethically permissible? *Family Practice* **18**, 511–515.

Medical Council of New Zealand (2006). *Sexual boundaries in the doctor–patient relationship: a resource for doctors*. Medical Council of New Zealand, Wellington, NZ. Available at http://www.mcnz.org.nz/portals/0/Guidance/Sexual_Boundaries.pdf (accessed 19 August 2008).

Pathe MT, Mullen PE and Purcell R (2002). Patients who stalk doctors: their motives and management. *Medical Journal of Australia* **176**, 335–338.

Rosendal M and Olesen F (2005). Management of medically unexplained symptoms. *British Medical Journal* **330**, 4–5

Sarkar SP (2004). Boundary violation and sexual exploitation in psychiatry and psychotherapy: a review. *Advance in Psychiatric Treatment* **10**, 312–320.

Schneider M and Phillips SP (1997). A qualitative study of sexual harassment of female doctors by patients. *Social Science & Medical* **45**, 669–676.

Smith RC, Lein C, Collins C, Lyles JS, Given B, Dwamena FC, Coffey J, Hodges A, Gardiner JC, Goddeeris J and Given W (2003). Treating patients with medically unexplained symptoms in primary care. *Journal General Internal Medicine* **18**, 478–489.

Spence SA (2005). Patients bearing gifts: are there strings attached? *British Medical Journal* **331**, 1527–1729.

Chapter 5

Confidentiality in general practice

Introduction

Joanna Silks has been Dr Mackenzie's patient, on and off, for many years. She has anxiety and depression that are related to childhood sexual abuse and a difficult relationship within her marriage. She and Dr Mackenzie have had a rather unusual relationship: periodically, Joanna gets angry with him and decides she doesn't want him to be her GP any more. She then attempts to seek out another GP, but she has always returned to see Dr Mackenzie.

This time, Joanna came with a range of symptoms that Dr Mackenzie thought were related to her ongoing distress, and he thought she might have irritable bowel syndrome. Despite his endeavours to convince her otherwise, she insisted on a referral to a surgeon. Dr Mackenzie was generally happy to comply with patient wishes in this kind of situation, but he thought the surgeon needed to know something of her background history. Accordingly, he included a note in his referral letter about her anxiety and depression.

At the St Andrews practice, practice referral letters are sent with the patient in a sealed envelope. Joanna opened the letter and read it. It was about her, so Dr Mackenzie didn't have any problems with her doing that. Joanna, however, didn't like being described as a patient with an 'emotional disorder'. She came back to see Dr Mackenzie and said 'No, I don't want this in the letter, but I still want the referral'. Dr Mackenzie rewrote the letter.

Dr Mackenzie didn't feel all that comfortable about leaving out what he thought was important background for the surgeon. On the basis of his history, examination and investigations he didn't believe that the referral was an appropriate referral anyway but, as he said to his partner, John, the next day, 'If a patient requests and insists on a referral, it is very hard not to refer'; and he felt that the surgeon would have wanted to know. He thought it would make the surgeon's job much easier; it would have allowed him

---

Case 5.1 *(continued)*

perhaps to ask questions in a way that would have explored some of the issues more effectively. Knowing Joanna, Dr Mackenzie suspected that if the surgeon had asked for the background, she would have denied it. He thought the surgeon probably worked it out anyhow, but he would have handled it better if he had access to something of what Dr Mackenzie knew about Joanna.

Maintaining patient confidentiality has a long and venerable history in medical practice. Many GPs will be familiar with the version in which the promise of confidentiality is found in the Hippocratic oath:

> Whatever, in connection with my professional practice, or not in connection with it, I see or learn, in the life of man, which ought not to be spoken abroad, I will not divulge, as reckoning that all such should be kept secret.

As an obligation on medical practitioners, it is also enshrined in more recent codes of ethics, including the British General Medical Council guidance (2004):

> Patients have a right to expect that information about them will be held in confidence by their doctors. Confidentiality is central to trust between doctors and patients. Without assurances about confidentiality, patients may be reluctant to give doctors the information they need in order to provide good care. If you are asked to provide information about patients you must:
>
> inform patients about the disclosure, or check that they have already received information about it;
>
> anonymise data where unidentifiable data will serve the purpose;
>
> be satisfied that patients know about disclosures necessary to provide their care, or for local clinical audit of that care, that they can object to these disclosures but have not done so;
>
> seek patients' express consent to disclosure of information, where identifiable data is needed for any purpose other than the provision of care or for clinical audit–save in the exceptional circumstances described in this booklet;
>
> keep disclosures to the minimum necessary; and
>
> keep up to date with and observe the requirements of statute and common law, including data protection legislation.

Codes of ethics in other countries provide similar guidance:

> Maintain your patient's confidentiality. Exceptions to this must be taken very seriously. They may include where there is a serious risk to the patient or another person, where required by law, where part of approved research, or where there are overwhelming societal interests.
>
> (Australian Medical Association 2004, 2006)

A doctor shall respect the principle of medical confidentiality and not disclose without a patient's consent, information obtained in confidence or in the course of attending to the patient. However, confidentiality is not absolute. It may be over-ridden by legislation, court orders or when the public interest demands disclosure of such information. An example is national disease registries which operate under a strict framework which safeguards medical confidentiality.

There may be other circumstances in which a doctor decides to disclose confidential information without a patient's consent. When he does this, he must be prepared to explain and justify his decision if asked to do so.

A doctor is expected to take steps to ensure that the means by which he communicates or stores confidential medical information about patients are secure and the information is not accessible to unauthorised persons. This is particularly relevant to sending or storing medical information by electronic means, via a website or by email.

(Singapore Medical Council 2007)

This chapter expands on the guidance offered above. What, exactly, is confidentiality? Why is it important? When, if ever, may or must a doctor breach confidentiality?

What is confidentiality?

Confidentiality is a duty: it is something doctors have a moral and, often, legal obligation to maintain for their patients. In general, the duty of confidentiality requires that doctors keep secret the information they are given by a patient and/or which they discover or learn about patients through their professional interactions. Patients can expect that:

- all information they disclose to the doctor will not be passed on to a third party without the express consent of the patient; and
- the doctor will take reasonable steps to protect the information collected from patients from access by third parties (Beauchamp and Childress 2001).

It is important to note a few things about this definition. First, patients can freely waive the right to confidentiality. If a patient authorizes release of information, it is not a violation of the duty of confidentiality to provide it to those to whom the patient has authorised the release. Had Joanna agreed to the disclosure to the surgeon of all aspects of her history, Dr Mackenzie could have passed that information on without a second thought.

Second, 'information' needs to be interpreted fairly broadly. It includes not only what the patient says, the findings on examination, results of tests and procedures, diagnoses and outcomes of treatment, but includes what the patient may unconsciously convey (for example, their emotional state) and the fact that the person has been a patient at all (Hamblin 1992).

Finally, the doctor's obligation to keep confidences relates not only to what he or she may consciously pass on to others about patients; it includes accidental and unwitting releases of information about patients. For example, leaving patient records open on the reception desk where visitors to the practice may see them, discussing a patient in an identifiable way with a colleague in a lift (Ubel 1995) and taking a call from or about a patient while another person is with you, may all be violations of the rule of confidentiality. These sorts of violations of confidentiality are particularly important in small, rural communities, where it is quite likely that people can piece together the identity of a patient from bits of information. Some of these inadvertent violations are unavoidable, but others are merely careless. Just because a doctor did not intend for sensitive information to reach the ears of others doesn't make it acceptable. 'I didn't think of it' is not a moral argument.

One of the most significant issues for confidentiality is the sharing of information about patients that goes on within health teams. In a world in which the one-to-one relationship between doctor and patient is often complicated by group practices, specialization, team management, quality assurance mechanisms and the like, it can be very difficult to uphold a promise of absolute confidentiality. It was his awareness of these practices that prompted Siegler in 1982 to suggest that confidentiality was a 'decrepit concept' that had past its prime.

Siegler and others may have been correct to be pessimistic about the future of confidentiality. Certainly, in the 25 years that have passed since his article, violations of confidentiality of the type he described have become increasingly common. However, the ubiquity of such breaches does not necessarily mean that they are justified. Justice Michael Kirby, for example, has argued for a renewed commitment to the value of confidentiality and careful review of any breaches (Kirby 1999). We still need to examine the ethical reasons for confidentiality and the situations in which breaches may be ethically acceptable.

Why is confidentiality important?

On a daily basis, we are surrounded by situations in which information about people is not kept confidential. The recent glut of reality TV shows bears witness to the extent to which some people are willing to live with little or no privacy. How can we justify a rule of confidentiality for general practitioners? What makes not keeping a confidence wrong?

Confidentiality is important for a number of reasons. Some of these reasons relate to what confidentiality can achieve for individual patients and the broader society. Other reasons focus on what confidentiality expresses–respect for patient autonomy and a promise kept with society. How these reasons function to justify the maintaining of confidentiality is important, not just as a matter of philosophical interest but particularly to help us work out what to do when we think breaches of confidentiality may be justified.

Confidentiality offers benefits for individual patients, both in terms of their likely usage of health services and the quality of care they may receive. Some patients may not seek medical care unless they are assured of confidentiality. For example, adolescent girls may be less likely to seek contraceptive advice if they know their parents may be told. People diagnosed with HIV may present later in their illness if there is mandatory reporting. Once in the consulting room, such patients will not be completely open and honest with their doctor unless they know that what is said in that room will be kept secret. There is a real limit to how well a doctor can diagnose, treat and care if patients provide only a partial account of themselves and their illnesses. The promise of confidentiality has an important bearing on the relationship of trust between individual doctors and patients.

Confidentiality in the doctor–patient relationship also has benefits beyond those that accrue to individual patients. Some people argue that an environment in which confidentiality is taken for granted is essential to provide the climate of trust and confidence that we need for any health care to be provided. Put another way, it would lead to poor outcomes for everyone if we did not have rules of confidentiality in medicine. Not only might individual patients suffer because of the reasons already outlined, but also the community would lose trust in the medical profession and in medical care. Doctors would not be able to do their jobs properly because they would never be sure that the information on which they were basing their decisions was accurate.

We do not necessarily know, in real life, whether confidentiality rules always increase the quality and outcomes of medical care. If you could show that the patient, their family or the community in general, would be better off if confidentiality were breached, then it might be acceptable not to keep a confidence. We will look at some reasons for breaching confidentiality below, but for now it sufficient to note that, regardless of how good or poor these utilitarian arguments for confidentiality are, there are other, deontologically based arguments that support a rule of confidentiality for doctors.

The first of these deontological arguments is that confidentiality is important because it expresses respect for patients' autonomy. We explore the notion of respect for autonomy in detail in Chapter 8. Here we merely note that respecting others' autonomy includes acknowledging that patients have aspects of their lives that they should be able to keep secret if they choose. It also means taking care to ensure that patients are not observed, touched or intruded upon without their consent. Some of us are more concerned about our privacy than others but, in our individualistic society, the right to be able to choose who has access to information about us is generally accorded a very high value. And doctors, by virtue of their professional work, often have access to highly personal, sometimes shameful and embarrassing, information, information that many people do not want revealed to a wider audience. When patients provide doctors with information, that information continues to belong to the patient and he or she can expect that the doctor will not pass on information about them to unauthorized others.

A final way to justify the rule of confidentiality is to see it as deriving from the obligation that all doctors have to keep faith with their community. The key idea here is the notion of keeping promises and commitments. How is keeping a promise or a commitment related to keeping information about patients confidential? After all, we don't make an explicit promise to each and every patient we see. However, there is a *social* expectation that doctors will keep information about patients secret. In a sense, when you become a doctor, you promise the community that you will keep the information patients give you confidential. Having made that promise, you 'no longer start from scratch in weighing the moral factors of a situation' (Bok 1983). You have already committed yourself to respect the confidentiality of the information you are given, so that divulging that information to other people is like breaking a promise. This type of argument helps to explain why we think it acceptable to tell others what our next door neighbour paid for his house or our views about the quality of work of the local plumber, even though it is unacceptable for doctors to chat about patients with a friend (Rhodes 2001).

We have set out four related reasons for why confidentiality is important. While these reasons offer powerful arguments for why we should not break the rule of confidentiality, it is very important to recognize that there are some circumstances in which it is permissible, and sometimes even necessary, on either moral or legal grounds, to breach confidentiality. The next section explores situations in which confidentiality can be a problem.

Cases in which maintaining confidentiality can be a problem

The primary obligation that general practitioners have to maintain confidentiality is simply stated. It is much harder to define those circumstances under which it is acceptable to break a confidence. In general, breaches of confidentiality fall into one of more of the following groups:

- situations in which we are unsure whether patients are in a position to decide for themselves;
- situations in which it seems to be in the best interests of the *patient* to break the rule of confidentiality; and/or

◆ situations in which it seems to be in the best interests of *others* to break the rule of confidentiality.

When patients may not be able to decide for themselves

Some of the most difficult cases are those in which the general practitioner is concerned that the patient is not really able to make a competent choice. For example, consider Dr McDonald's position here:

Case 5.2

Mrs Logan, an 85-year-old woman, is brought to see her GP, Dr Fiona McDonald, by her next door neighbours. Mrs Logan's neighbours explain that they became concerned after they noticed Mrs Logan had not collected her mail for two days. They found Mrs Logan in bed with sheets stained with vomitus and faeces. When they could not reach her daughter, Lucinda, by telephone, they decided to bring Mrs Logan to the surgery themselves.

When Dr McDonald questions Mrs Logan, she seems confused and she is vague about what has happened to her in the last two days. After examining her, Dr McDonald decides to admit Mrs Logan to hospital. She explains to Mrs Logan what she is going to do and that she will ring her daughter to let her know what has happened. Mrs Logan says quite clearly that she doesn't want Lucinda to know; she doesn't want to bother her daughter who is 'busy with the grandchildren'.

Dr McDonald is surprised by this response; Lucinda usually accompanies her mother when she comes for her regular checkups and Mrs Logan has always seemed happy to involve her daughter in her medical care.

In this situation Dr McDonald is probably not sure that she needs to respect Mrs Logan's apparent desire for confidentiality. One of the reasons Dr McDonald is unsure is because the foundations on which the promise of confidentiality is built seem to be in doubt here. First, Dr McDonald is reasonably confident that Mrs Logan is not functioning as an autonomous decision-maker. Her response seems most out of character with her usual behaviour; it seems that Mrs Logan's medical condition is clearly influencing her awareness and understanding of her situation. Confidentiality may be justified by the principle of respect for autonomy, but when we have doubts about the autonomy of the patient, that justification can seem rather weak. For this reason, it may be permissible for Dr McDonald to contact Mrs Logan's daughter.

Mrs Logan's circumstance is not the only one in which general practitioners can face questions about confidentiality and competence. The care of children and adolescents, and people with psychiatric illness, mental disability and drug and alcohol abuse can all create situations in which the capacity of a patient to make an autonomous decision is in doubt.

When breaching confidentiality may be in the patient's best interests

Even if Dr McDonald had no concerns about Mrs Logan's competence, she might be tempted to breach confidentiality for a second reason. Dr McDonald may wonder whether keeping this secret will be in Mrs Logan's best interests. She may believe that Mrs Logan will improve more rapidly if she has the support and help of a family who have already shown themselves to be genuinely concerned for her wellbeing.

Dr McDonald's reasons are similar to the reasons Dr Mackenzie might have offered for breaching confidentiality. When Dr Mackenzie included a comment about Joanna's psychosocial history in his referral letter, he was doing what he thought would be in her best interests. He naturally included in the letter those aspects of Joanna's medical history that he considered relevant for the management of her current condition. He believed that Joanna's psychosocial history was important; he probably also knew, given her concern not to be described as someone with an 'emotional disorder', that it was unlikely Joanna would tell the surgeon herself about her anxiety and depression.

A lot turns, in these two cases, on how confident the general practitioners can be that their judgement of the patients' best interests is the correct one. The interpretation of patients' best interests is a complex moral issue that we discuss in detail in the next chapter. Here we note only that, while it is true that more openness about the patient's condition can often have significant benefits for patients—through more accurate diagnosis, more appropriate treatment or better support in distressing situations—it is also true that patients do not always see such things in the same light as their doctors do. For example, Dr McDonald may only see those aspects of Lucinda's relationship with her mother that she wishes the GP to see. In private, Lucinda may be a reluctant support for her mother. Dr Mackenzie's frequent contact with people in psychological distress may lead him to understate the stigmatizing effect of mental illness for Joanna. There may be a conflict here between a justification for confidentiality that is based on privacy, autonomy and promise-keeping and one that is based on the best interests of the patient. This is one of the central issues for medical ethics, and we return to it again in Chapters 6 and 8.

When breaching confidentiality may be in the best interests of others

The final group of problems for confidentiality relates to situations in which GPs think that other people may be harmed or, at least, not helped if they do not break a confidence. The following case provides an example of just such an ethical dilemma.

Case 5.3

One evening Margaret presents to the surgery with an obvious case of delirium tremens due to acute alcohol withdrawal. Despite being a well-known patient, this is the first time that Dr McDonald is aware that Margaret has an alcohol dependency problem, and that she usually drinks half a bottle of vodka per day while working as a registered child-minder caring for children in her own home. The doctor advises admission but Margaret refuses as she has children booked in for the next day.

Dr McDonald is concerned that Margaret is intoxicated whilst caring for children, and that the children may be at risk of harm because of this. Margaret promises to stop drinking.

Over the next few months Margaret appears to be refraining from alcohol. In the meantime, Dr McDonald has attempted to clarify the ethical and legal situation. Her Medical Defence Union has advised her that if the patient has given her word that she is not drinking, then Dr McDonald has no right to breach confidentiality on the grounds of possible danger to the children in her care. The opinion of the defence union is that the medical registration authority would consider striking off Dr McDonald if she breached confidentiality and the patient complained.

David Grainger, one of Dr McDonald's partners, feels very strongly that Dr McDonald should notify social services, using the 'What would the papers say?' argument. What would the papers say if there was a fire and a child was injured as a result of the child-minder's intoxication and Dr McDonald had not acted, despite her knowledge of the danger?

Social services, contacted by telephone with a general inquiry, were not interested in the situation as their resources are stretched to the limit dealing with actual cases of child abuse: 'Children are looked after by drunk parents all the time and we don't interfere'.

A few months later, Margaret is obviously drinking again. Dr McDonald urges her to stop work. Margaret says that she will contact the child-minder's registration authority and inform them that she is no longer active.

Case 5.3 *(continued)*

However, suspension of work is voluntary, and child-minders can recommence work whenever they wish without giving a reason for their break and without any re-registration processes.

Dr McDonald contacts a friend in social services and explains the nature of the problem. She is concerned that the voluntary nature of the arrangement may not hold, and that Margaret may start caring for children again at any time. The social worker advises calling the registration authority.

Dr McDonald calls the registration authority and asks to know the status of Margaret's registration. The authority wants to know why. Dr McDonald replies that she cannot give the reason. After some further conversation, the registration authority ask whether it will be satisfactory if they ask Margaret to return her registration certificate, which means that she will require a full healthcare check prior to become registered again. Dr McDonald says, 'Yes'.

This dilemma caused much anxiety for Dr McDonald who felt very strongly that if she did not act, children were potentially at risk. She felt that there was no one to consult over a problem of this kind, and that the attitude of the defence union was less than helpful.

In contrast to other situation in which GPs do have a duty to notify of possible danger to the public (e.g. bus driver with epilepsy), there are no procedures for notifying about problems with child-minders, despite their occupational responsibilities towards the children they care for. Given the vulnerability of children, and the fact that the children themselves are not likely to notice anything amiss in the behaviour of their carer, what should Dr McDonald's responsibilities be in this case?

It is worth noting, at the beginning of our discussion of this case, that it takes place in a particular legal and social context. There are a small number of situations in which GPs are required, by law, to provide information about patients to third parties, usually to a clearly specified organization, such as the police or the health department. Although the precise requirements will vary from country to country, in general GPs are required to pass on information about patients, without their consent, if necessary, when:

- reporting notifiable diseases, including sexually transmitted diseases;
- notifying births and deaths (including underlying cause of death);
- there are concerns about a patient's fitness to be granted a driver's licence; or
- when child abuse is suspected or confirmed.

Some of these situations are relatively straightforward. The decision to breach or not breach confidentiality often becomes a non-decision when the law *requires* such breaches. For example, death certificates are legally required to be completed honestly and fully, to the best of the doctor's knowledge and belief. Sometimes, if the cause of death is thought to be potentially stigmatizing, such as suicide or HIV/AIDS, the relatives of the deceased may request that the cause of death is not written on the certificate. Such requests may be very understandable to the GP, but there are other factors to consider. Death certificates are important epidemiological data; their usefulness depends upon their accuracy. The public duty to provide accurate information outweighs the individual interests of the bereaved. In addition, inaccurate death certificates may be used for fraudulent insurance claims.

The fact that the law does require GPs to break confidences in some situations is of relevance to the ethical issues at hand here. Waller puts it well when he notes that, in situations in which passing on information to others is mandated, 'the legislature has, presumably, there done the business of balancing competing interests; medical confidentiality has been outweighed by the public interest in the administration of justice, or the community's general health, or the prevention of serious crime' (Waller 1993, p.198).

Waller's point is that, in these circumstances, we could, if we were inclined to follow the argument through, justify breaches of confidentiality because other people's interests outweigh individuals' concerns to protect their privacy. The 'other' interests relate to two groups. First, there are interests that can be linked to identifiable individuals. For example, GPs may become aware of inherited diseases, such as Huntington's disease, that are carried by some members of a family and of which other members of the family are unaware. They may be torn between wanting to respect a patient's desire for secrecy and realizing that other family members should have access to relevant information before they make important decisions about careers, marriage and child-bearing. As genetic testing becomes more common, such situations are likely to arise more often (Lucassen and Parker 2004).

In the Tarasoff case, which came before the Californian Supreme Court in 1976, the failure by a psychologist to breach confidentiality had tragic consequences for an identifiable individual. The Tarasoff case concerned a university student who confided to the psychologist treating him at a university counselling service that he intended to kill his girl friend, Tatiana Tarasoff. The young woman was clearly identifiable. The psychologist was concerned enough to attempt to have the student committed for psychiatric evaluation. His efforts were unsuccessful and the patient was released from temporary police custody and ended his therapy. Neither the psychologist, nor the police, made any attempt to warn Tatiana, or her family, that her life might be in danger. Two months later, the student killed Tatiana. Her family sued the psychologist and the University for damages and the Supreme Court of California held that both were liable, on the grounds that the psychologist had a duty to attempt to prevent harm to an identifiable individual and that there was clear evidence that Tatiana was in grave danger.

The second group of interests are those that cannot necessarily be linked to identifiable people. In these cases, we may not be able to tie the benefits to be gained (or the harms to be prevented) by breaching confidentiality to recognizable individuals. It may be, rather, that we think the breach is warranted on the grounds of benefits to society as a whole or to particular groups in society. The rationale for mandatory reporting of sexually transmitted diseases to the health department, informing road traffic authorities that a patient is not fit to drive or reporting patients whom one suspects of terrorist activity, falls into this category. In the second and third cases, particularly, it is almost impossible to identify precisely the people who might be harmed if an unfit driver continued to drive or if a patient did indeed carry out a terrorist act.

Such situations are interesting from a public policy point of view, and they are similar in type to the ethical dilemma that Dr McDonald faces in our third case. However, they do not raise the acute problems that Dr McDonald experiences. Dr McDonald's moral dilemma is complicated because her attempts to create some certainty for herself have, so far, been ineffective.

Dr McDonald's unsuccessful search for legal and regulatory clarity is probably not an isolated incident. These cases are immensely difficult and the law does not always offer GPs clear guidance on what they should do (Hamblin 1992; Waller 1993). In recent times, the courts have had to consider a number of cases in which a breach of confidentiality, on grounds of the public interest, was the central issue. Fortunately or unfortunately, the courts have arrived at conclusions that suggest only that 'there is very little certainty as to how a court will determine the operation of the public interest exception in any given case' (Hamblin 1992, p.430.) In this environment, what can Dr McDonald do, and why should she do it?

As she thinks about these issues, it may be helpful for Dr McDonald to attempt to clarify the *size* and the *risk* of harm to the children in Margaret's care. She may also wish to think about the extent to which whatever she does will actually prevent the harm from occurring. Put another way, Dr McDonald might ask herself: 'Is there a *substantial* risk of *serious avoidable* harm to others in this situation?' (Beauchamp and Childress 2001, pp.308–309). Let's look at each of the issues identified in this question in turn.

First, what is the size or seriousness of the harm that might befall others? Is someone's life in danger? Or, is it rather that a third party will merely experience minor, self-limiting harm if the doctor does not breach confidentiality? In general, the more serious the harms that may arise if a GP does not intervene, the greater the likelihood that the GP's intervention can be regarded as ethically acceptable. In this case, the harms that might befall these children are variable. At one end of the spectrum, Margaret's drinking may mean only that the children do not get fed on time, or that they spend all day watching television. If these were the extent of the harms likely to befall the children in Margaret's care, Dr McDonald would probably have little justification for interfering. After all, as the social services office implies, many children are not adequately cared for, but society rarely intervenes to rescue them. In this case, though, there are other, far more serious, consequences that may arise if Margaret drinks to excess while caring for children. Dr McDonald's colleague has already raised the possibility of a fire; one could equally imagine a child running on to a road, injuring himself in a fall or drowning in a bath. Any of these events would have serious consequences for the children.

The seriousness of the harm is not the only issue to take into account. The second component to our question relates to the size of the risk or the probability that the harm will occur. How likely is it that the harm will actually eventuate? Again, the higher the probability or risk of harm, the greater the obligation on the part of the GP to intervene. In Tatiana Tarasoff's case, the psychologist was concerned enough about the likelihood that his patient would act on his stated intention that he sought to have him detained. He considered that the risk of harm to Tatiana was quite high. This will not always be the case and there will be situations in which the GP may realize that the risk of harm to others is actually relatively low. Dr McDonald's dilemma falls somewhere in between and she may require more information to assess the risks accurately. For example, she may need to assess how likely it is that Margaret will take up work again. Obviously, the risk of harm to children evaporates when Margaret is not child-minding. But, will Dr McDonald be in a position to know if Margaret goes back to work? Beyond these considerations, some people might argue that the risk of calamitous events here is actually quite low, and perhaps not all that much higher than the background level of risk for all children.

Finally, Dr McDonald will need to consider the extent to which whatever she chooses or is able to do can somehow change things for the children Margaret cares for. Dr McDonald's actions so far have had some impact. However, it is still possible that, despite her intervention, Margaret may continue to do informal, unregistered child-minding. If Dr McDonald decides that breaching confidentiality by informing the registration authority is not really going to change things, then she ought to reconsider whether informing the authority at all has been worthwhile. Alternatively, she may need to think about other actions she can take that are more likely to protect the children from harm. For example, she could take the drastic step of trying to inform parents that their child-minder was drinking heavily while caring for their children.

When Dr McDonald has considered these issues, she still has to weigh the harms and/or benefits for the children against the need to respect Margaret's confidences and to act in ways that are in Margaret's best interests. This balancing, and the decisions that follow from it, will always be difficult.

Conclusion

In this chapter, we have explored the ethical issues that arise from the obligation to respect confidences. Although confidentiality is not an absolute duty, in most cases, breaching confidentiality requires a heavy burden of proof. Reaching an ethically acceptable decision will often hinge, in large part, on weighing the relative merits of patients' best interests and the duty to respect the autonomy of patients.

References

Australian Medical Association (2004, 2006) *AMA code of ethics.* Available at http://www.ama.com.au/web.nsf/doc/WEEN-6VQ2NX/$file/ AMA_Code_of_Ethics__2004._Editorially_Revised_2006.pdf (accessed 25 August 2008).

Beauchamp TL and Childress JF (2001). *Principles of biomedical ethics* (5th edn) Oxford University Press. New York, 303–312.

Bok S (1983). The limits of confidentiality. *Hastings Center Report* **13**, 24–31.

General Medical Council (2004). *Guidance on good practice. confidentiality.* General Medical Council, London. Available at http://www.gmc-uk.org/guidance/ current/library/confidentiality.asp#28 (accessed 25 August 2008).

Hamblin J (1992). Confidentiality, public interest and the health professional's duty of care. *Australian Health Review* **15**, 422–434.

The Hippocratic Oath. Available at http://classics.mit.edu/Hippocrates/hippooath.htm (accessed 25 August 2008).

Kirby M (1999). Privacy protection–a new beginning. In *Proceedings of the 21st International Conference on Privacy and Personal Data Protection.* Hong Kong, 13–14 September 1999. Hong Kong: Office of the Privacy Commissioner for Personal Data, 8.

Lucassen A and Parker M (2004). Confidentiality and serious harm in genetics–preserving the confidentiality of one patient and preventing harm to relatives. *European Journal of Human Genetics* **12**, 93–97.

Rhodes R (2001). Understanding the trusted doctor and constructing a theory of bioethics. *Theoretical Medicine and Bioethics* **22**, 493–504.

Siegler M (1982). Confidentiality in medicine: a decrepit concept. *New England Journal of Medicine* **307**, 1518–1521.

Singapore Medical Council (2007). *Ethical code and ethical guideline.* Available at http://www.smc.gov.sg/html/1150880218803.html (accessed 25 August 2008).

Ubel PA, Zell MM, Miller DJ, Fischer GS, Peters-Stefani D and Arnold RM (1995). Elevator talk: observational study of inappropriate comments in a public space. *American Journal of Medicine* **99**, 190–194.

Waller L (1993). Secrets revealed: the limits of medical confidence. *Journal of Contemporary Health Law and Policy* **9**, 183–210.

Further guidance on confidentiality

American Medical Association. *AMA code of ethics principles of medical ethics.* Available at http://www.ama-assn.org/ama/pub/category/2498.html (accessed 25 August 2008).

Canadian Medical Association. *CMA code of ethics.* Available at http://www.cma.ca/index.cfm/ci_id/53556/la_id/1.htm (accessed 25 August 2008).

General Medical Council (United Kingdom). *Good medical practice. Confidentiality: protecting and providing information.* Available at http://www.gmc-uk.org/guidance/current/library/confidentiality.asp (accessed 25 August 2008).

Medical Council (Ireland). *Guide to ethical conduct and behaviour* (6thedn). PDF dwnload available at http://www.medicalcouncil.ie/professional/ethics.asp (accessed 25 August 2008).

New Zealand Medical Association. *NZMA code of ethics.* Available at http://www.nzma.org.nz/about/ethics.html (accessed 25 August 2008).

World Medical Association. *International code of medical ethics.* Available at http://www.wma.net/e/policy/c8.htm (accessed 25 August 2008).

Chapter 6

Beneficence or does the doctor know best?

Introduction

Case 6.1

Sibyl Price presents to Dr Jeremy Chu with tiredness. On examination, Dr Chu detects enlarged cervical and axillary nodes. The nodes are rubbery rather than tender. Dr Chu's first impression is that this could be leukaemia or lymphoma, with viral infection as a secondary diagnosis. He arranges blood tests without explaining to Mrs Price the likely causes of her illness or the specific investigations.

If we asked Dr Chu what he is doing, he may well reply that he is acting in the best interests of his patient. What does this mean? In our example, Dr Chu might say that he is medically trained and has expertise in formulating symptoms and signs into a working diagnosis, and then confirming this with relevant investigations. Performing the blood tests is a way of checking the accuracy of his working diagnosis, and it is his job to know which tests to perform and how to interpret the results. As the patient has no training in medicine, there is no point in discussing with her which tests to do.

Dr Chu might also say that the woman is feeling unwell, she is anxious as well as tired, and that it is not fair to burden her with possible diagnoses until the clinical situation is clearer. He might say that it is part of the doctor's responsibilities to keep silent about all the possible diagnoses, especially potentially serious ones, and that the patient expects him to sort out the problem and then tell her, rather than involving her in the fear and uncertainty of tentative diagnoses.

He might also say that part of the therapeutic power of medicine is related to his expertise and willingness to take responsibility, and that the patient feels better if her care is provided by a doctor who takes charge. The patient's confidence may be undermined if the doctor does not act in a directive way that indicates he is in control of the situation. Later in the chapter we shall analyse these justifications in detail, but first we shall examine the ethical obligation that underlies the idea of acting in the best interests of the patient.

The principle of beneficence

The principle of beneficence imposes a duty upon doctors to act always for the good of their patients. This is the very heart of morality–one of the ways we judge the goodness or badness of an action is by asking the question: Are we trying to help or harm? We can think of this in two ways, in terms of underlying motive, and in terms of the actual effects or consequences of our actions. In medicine it is difficult to be certain that our actions will always lead to good outcomes; given the vagaries of disease processes and treatment responses we cannot guarantee this in advance. However, we can examine our motives and ask whether our action is motivated by the aim of benefiting the patient. In general, medical practice is considered inherently beneficent, as it promises assistance to the sick or injured, aiming to ameliorate or prevent the harms of ill health. (See also Chapter 13 on the virtuous practitioner.)

As an ethical principle, beneficence is central to most codes of professional ethics, going all the way back to Hippocrates. The Hippocratic Oath says that 'I will prescribe regimens for the good of my patients according to my ability and my judgement and never do harm to anyone' and 'In every house where I come I will enter only for the good of my patients' (Wikipedia 2008). Modern codes take a similar line. For example, the first of the duties of doctors listed by the General Medical Council in the UK is to 'make the care of your patient your first concern' (General Medical Council 2006).

The Hippocratic Oath picks out two important aspects of beneficence. The first is to do with using medical expertise to help rather than harm the patient. Historically, the medical knowledge that doctors have is specialized and generally unavailable to patients. Although increased access to medical information provided via the internet is changing this balance in various ways, patients still look to their doctors for expert knowledge. As this knowledge could be used either to heal or damage patients, accepting the obligation of beneficence harnesses that power for patients' good and limits the potential for harm. The duty to use medical knowledge for good rather than for harm is so foundational that it is taken for granted. Only when there are breaches of this duty, such as using medical expertise to torture prisoners or murder patients, are we shocked into reflecting as to why such actions are so reprehensible. Using medical knowledge and expertise intentionally to harm people violates the fundamental principle of beneficence.

The second part of the quote from the Hippocratic oath states that 'I will enter only for the good of my patient'. This refers to the privileges accorded to doctors, and the uses to which they may be put. Doctors collect private information about patients and have extensive physical access to their patients. Both of these privileges could be abused; for example, by gossiping about a patient's diagnosis or prognosis, or by performing unnecessary breast and genital examinations. The moral requirement to use these privileges only for the good of the patient aims to prevent actions performed for reasons other than the patient's good, such as personal gratification.

As the expression of a moral ideal, acting for the benefit of others is straightforward; difficulties arise, however, when we try to determine what kind of obligations should guide our actions in general practice. In general, there are three kinds of problems when we try to work out what it means in practice to act for the good of patients. The first is working out what we mean by the patient's best interests, the second is treading the fine line between beneficence and paternalism, and the third concerns finding out just what is the medical good for this particular patient.

Acting in the patient's best interests

In some situations, it is very straightforward to say what acting in the patient's best interests might be. If we think back to Trevor's case in Chapter 3, it was in his interests to be treated immediately for meningitis. Similarly, a person with severe chest pain has their interests served by prompt investigation to confirm or exclude myocardial infarction. For many consultations in general practice, there is an obvious health problem for which it is in the patient's best interests to receive definitive advice or treatment.

Yet often things are not so straightforward, and this can be especially the case in general practice where there can be conflicts between the health interests of a person and other important interests that the person might have. Patients visiting GPs are not as removed from their usual daily lives as patients in hospital, making it imperative to take account of wider issues when considering the patient's best interests. There may, for example, be tensions between a person's health interests and their employment interests.

Case 6.2

Barry Black is an apprentice plumber who works for a fairly unsympathetic boss. He presents to Dr Singh with a badly bruised and sprained right wrist. The injury occurred when a piece of equipment broke while ditch digging. Dr Singh arranges for an X-ray to exclude fracture, and then splints the wrist. Dr Singh advises two weeks rest, followed by physiotherapy. Mr Black is reluctant to be signed off for this long, as he cannot afford the drop in income, and he knows that his boss will be angry if this is recorded as a work-related injury.

Barry's interest in maintaining his income and staying on the right side of his boss is in direct conflict with his medical interests. Given the medical advice, it is then up to him to work out how to balance these competing interests. Duties to family members are another source of competing interests. What of a woman with severe chest pain, who is single and caring for a daughter with Down syndrome, who does not wish to go to hospital for investigations or admission because this will leave her daughter with no carer? Again there is a conflict between what is medically best for the person in terms of her health interests, and what may be best overall, given all of the interests in her life.

These conflicts are common in general practice, because general practice takes place within the community where GPs are constantly faced with the reality and importance of their patients' interests over and above any immediate health problems. In secondary and tertiary care, the health problem can be so urgent or overwhelming that the patient's interests have shrunk to coincide with their health interests. If the woman with chest pain has a heart attack, all of her interests rely upon successful treatment for the heart attack. Such urgent situations are rare in general practice. Commonly GPs have the sometimes difficult task of determining the importance of health amongst the wider interests of their patients.

Sometimes it is hard for doctors to appreciate the other interests that patients have; medical training tends to foster powerful normative views about health and illness, so that doctors may feel very strongly about what the right thing to do is, with regard to health. This can lead to absurdity when carried to extremes.

Case 6.3

Mrs Stirling is a fit 85-year-old woman. She has some minor arthritis in her hands, for which she takes anti-inflammatories. When attending the Gordon Road Practice for a repeat prescription, Dr Grainger urged Mrs Stirling to

> **Case 6.3** *(continued)*
>
> have her cholesterol checked. Her cholesterol level was found to be slightly elevated, and Dr Grainger advised Mrs Stirling to cut down on her dairy products. Her sole dairy intake was a nightly mug of a malted milk drink, which she duly sacrificed for the sake of her cholesterol level.
>
> Mrs Stirling was grateful to Dr Grainger for identifying this problem and alerting her to the dangers of drinking milk.

In this case, Dr Grainger used a narrow medical view of the patient's interests, understood solely in terms of serum lipid levels. On the basis of this, he prescribed changes in behaviour with no discussion of the actual risks for Mrs Stirling of continuing her nightly mug of milk, or the effect of this sacrifice upon her sleep patterns or overall enjoyment in life. General practice prides itself on taking a holistic view of patients; if this is to be taken seriously, GPs must take a wide rather than a narrow view of patients' interests when they consider their obligations to act beneficently.

Beneficence and paternalism

The duty to act beneficently applies to all doctors but, as we have said, the scope of patients' interests can vary by specialty and circumstances. In general practice, patients may present with a wide range of physical, mental and social problems, so that to respond competently and comprehensively, GPs must use a broad understanding of best interests (Christie and Hoffmaster 1986; Rogers 1999). At times, beneficence takes the form of taking charge of the patient, leading us into the sometimes tricky region where morally justifiable beneficence may slip over into morally questionable paternalism.

What is paternalism and why is it morally questionable? Paternalism involves forms of what we may call 'caring control': acting for the good of another person, but in a way that disregards the wishes of the recipient. This is the moral problem–paternalists act for the good of patients without taking any account of what the patient might want for themselves. Paternalistic actions can range from non-intrusive, such as offering advice, through to concerted efforts to influence behaviour or actions that restrict freedom (Häyry 1998). The key feature that distinguishes paternalism from beneficence is that paternalistic actions do not take account of, and may override, a person's expressed wishes or desires. Although all paternalistic actions should be motivated by the welfare or good of the recipient, not all of them can be morally justified, especially where the action involves overriding the autonomy of the person involved.

Paternalistic actions occur across a spectrum. At one end, health education and public health advertisements are examples of soft paternalism because they attempt to influence people's behaviour, irrespective of whether or not people want the information or to have their behaviour changed. This is soft paternalism because it uses persuasion rather than stronger methods. At the other end of the spectrum, hard paternalism does involve controlling people's actions; for example, by lying, concealing information or compelling treatment. Hard paternalism is further defined in terms of being either 'weak' or 'strong'. Weak paternalism occurs when a person is controlled in some way, but that person is not fully capable of making their own decisions for reasons such as mental incapacity, lack of knowledge, lack of control over their actions, or acting under undue influence. In all of these situations, the paternalism may be justified if the action is necessary to prevent harm and if the person's capacity to make decisions really is impaired. Examples of weak medical paternalism include detention of a psychotic patient at risk of harming herself, vaccinating an unwilling child, or treating a patient with anorexia nervosa.

In contrast, strong paternalism occurs when there are attempts to control people who *are* capable of making their own decisions. For example, admitting an elderly but competent patient to a nursing home against his wishes, or refusing to inform a woman with an unwanted pregnancy about legal abortion services, are strongly paternalistic, because in both cases, the person involved is capable of choosing their own course of action. The crucial point here is that, although the doctor may think that they are acting for the good of the patient, there is no element of consent and the patient is not respected as person who is capable of making decisions.

There is debate about when and if strong paternalism can be justified. Childress (2007) offers a series of conditions for justifying strong paternalism in healthcare (see Box 6.1). These conditions provide a useful framework for thinking about particular situations, but it may be tempting for the doctor with paternalistic tendencies to answer 'Yes' to all of them without fully considering the alternatives or taking account of how the patient may feel about the proposed benefits and the impact of having their wishes overridden.

What of Mrs Price and Dr Chu? Dr Chu's decision not to discuss the reasons for the tests was paternalistic because he felt that he was acting for her good, without offering Mrs Price the chance to receive more information or to decline particular tests. He acted for her good without taking account of her wishes in the matter. There was no apparent reason to doubt her capacity to understand information or participate in decisions, making this an example of strong paternalism. Could this be justified using the criteria in Box 6.1? If we assume that he withheld information because he did not want to worry

Box 6.1 Conditions for strong paternalism

There is a risk to the patient of serious and preventable harm.

The paternalistic action will probably prevent the harm.

The paternalistic action is necessary to prevent the harm.

The risks of the intervention are outweighed by the anticipated benefits to the patient.

The anticipated benefits outweigh the harm caused by not respecting the autonomy of the patient.

The paternalistic action is the least restrictive alternative necessary to avoid the harm (adapted from Childress 2007, p. 225).

her, it is hard to see how this could be justified unless we take her worry to be a 'serious and preventable harm'. Perhaps he knows her to be an extremely anxious person who has declined similar information in the past on the grounds that she finds it too distressing to know about possible diagnoses, and only wishes to know once the diagnosis is definite. But, unless this was the case, the paternalism seems unjustified on that ground alone.

Why might he act like this? As discussed above, there is often an assumption that the person acting paternalistically is wiser, more knowledgeable or more experienced than the person they act for, and this justifies taking charge. In medicine there is a temptation to move from the fact that doctors are more expert than patients, to the assumption that this expertise can justify making decisions on patients' behalf. Some patients may expect or welcome doctors taking charge, but it is unacceptably paternalistic if the GP assumes that they know how to benefit the patient without finding out what the patient would actually prefer. Assuming that the patient is not capable of understanding medical information or deciding 'not to worry' the person with information because the doctor thinks that this may be burdensome are both forms of unacceptable paternalism.

As well as overt paternalism achieved by controlling patient's behaviour, paternalistic attitudes can be harmful to patients by undermining their confidence in their abilities to participate in decision-making. Paternalistic attitudes are sometimes pervasive, conveyed through language in phrases such as 'You don't need to worry about this', or by condescending or overbearing behaviour (Downie and Calman 1994).

Medicine and paternalism

Claims of paternalism have often been levelled at medical practitioners. Why might this be so? Dr Chu offered three familiar reasons to explain his paternalism (Sherwin 1992).

Box 6.2 Common explanations for paternalism

1. The vulnerability of the sick: ill people may be anxious or stressed by their illness, making them potentially unfit to make decisions, so that it better for doctors, who are unaffected by the illness, to make the decisions.

2. Medical expertise: doctors are the experts, so this makes them the right ones to make decisions for patients.

3. Medical confidence and the placebo effect: unless doctors are confident and decisive in telling patients what to do, they will lose the healing power associated with patients having faith in their doctors.

In the following section we discuss these reasons in relation to general practice.

The vulnerability of the sick

Are general practice patients too ill to discuss relevant information or make decisions? In some situations (for example, unconscious patients) this is the case, and of course the GP should take responsibility for making decisions in that patient's best interests. Other forms of illness, even quite minor illness, can make a person feel fearful, tired, less capable or not wanting to be bothered with decisions, and this may be accompanied by a desire to be cared for. This, however, does not always translate into a desire for a paternalistic GP. It may be helpful to identify two separate activities here. The first is to do with giving information and the second is to do with making decisions. These are often run together, but either information and/or inclusion in decision-making may be withheld by doctors for paternalistic reasons.

Patients who feel ill may not want to be faced with medical decisions, but they may welcome information and explanations about their situation. Of course, judgement must come into this, and part of the skill of general practice lies in knowing the patient and knowing how much information they usually prefer. Paternalism creeps in when there is a unilateral decision by the GP that the patient does not need to know or would be better off not knowing.

What if the patient is faced with a serious diagnosis? Are they still able to take in information and make important decisions? Serious diagnoses can be devastating, accompanied by fear, grief and misery. This can impair a person's immediate capacity for decision-making. It would be naive to assume that a person can be given a diagnosis of lymphoma or breast cancer and then immediately be able to make important decisions. But usually there is no need for this kind of speed. Most medical decisions are not urgent; there is time to face the diagnosis, and talk about the patient's beliefs and wishes. This is especially the case in general practice, which offers the opportunity for patients to return after an initial diagnosis, to provide more information and to discuss the options.

The desire to spare patients uncertainty and fear can lead to paternalism. However, a paternalistic approach in this situation blocks the opportunity to discover the nature of the fears, and to sort out with the patient which fears are justified and to deal appropriately with those that are not. Ethically, it is preferable to discuss the patient's fears, so that a perhaps overwhelming fear of the unknown becomes replaced with fear of something more circumscribed and manageable. This approach supports the patient's capacity for future decision-making, and also reduces the perceived need for paternalism.

In many general practice consultations, patients are not ill. Chronic disease management, vaccinations, cervical smears or blood pressure checks, issuing various certificates, and follow-up consultations, all involve patients who are very much their usual, everyday selves, rather than ill or fearful. This means that it is relatively rare in general practice that paternalism can be grounded in an appeal to the patient's vulnerability.

Medical expertise

The second reason that is often offered for paternalism is that medical decision-making requires the medical expertise (scientific or technical knowledge) that is acquired through medical education. As doctors are the ones with this expertise, they are in the best position to know what is best for patients. The assumption here is that medical decisions are mainly scientific/technical in nature. However, many of the decisions that occur in general practice are not like this. For example, if a patient consults with lateral epicondylitis (tennis elbow), there are various treatment options, such as topical non-steroidal anti-inflammatory drugs, corticosteroid injection, physical therapies or surgery. The patient needs access to some technical information in order to make a decision, but the decision itself is not technical as it cannot properly be answered on purely technical grounds. The answer depends on the values the patient puts upon various factors, such as their level of pain and incapacity, their dissatisfaction with current therapy, the need to remain at work, their inclination to take risks or their capacity to access the various therapies. Of course there are situations in which doctors do know best in a straightforward sense—for example, which drug to prescribe, if drug therapy is preferred, or what kind of operation to perform, if there is a decision to proceed with surgery—but situations with a single technical solution are the exception rather than the rule in general practice.

One way of thinking about these issues is in terms of domains of expertise. This approach recognizes that most decisions in general practice require the expertise of both patient and GP. Medical expertise is important, in interpreting symptoms, developing and confirming diagnoses, and outlining the options for management. The patient needs this expertise to understand their problem and to decide about management. But medical expertise alone is not enough to reach an optimal decision; the patient also has expertise that she brings to the consultation. She is the one who knows how the problem is affecting her and how serious it is. She is also the expert as far as knowing what kind of management options will be acceptable or possible for her. Thinking about both the patient's and the GP's expertise in an explicit way helps to ensure that they both have the best possible understanding of the patient's interests and how these can be furthered. The two domains of expertise are complementary, and both are necessary for a holistic understanding of the patient's interests (Rogers 1999).

Medical confidence, communication and the placebo effect

A third explanation for paternalism revolves around the idea that it is important for doctors to act confidently, as faith in the doctor is good for patients. If the doctor is positive about, and the patient believes in, the likely successful outcomes of the treatment, this may contribute to the success of the treatment. The mechanisms for this are unclear but seem to be related in a specific way to communication styles and, more broadly, to the placebo effect. Two studies from general practice seem to demonstrate the beneficial effects of medical confidence. In the studies, one group of patients received a directive or positive style of consultation, and these patients were more satisfied, and some had significantly swifter symptom resolution than patients who received a negative or non-directive style of consultation (Thomas 1987; Savage and Armstrong 1990). More recent work appears to support the potential benefits of a positive approach in terms of decreased symptom burden (Little *et al.* 2001).

It is not clear from the available research whether the beneficial effects come from the positive promotion of the treatment or the elimination of uncertainty through this positive attitude. There has been a widely shared assumption that the disclosure of uncertainty is a bad thing for patients, and that uncertainty decreases doctors' effectiveness as healers (Katz 1984; Christie and

Hoffmaster 1986). Do patients really wish for certainty when they see a GP, or is it GPs who feel uncomfortable admitting or explaining or tolerating uncertainty? Not knowing a definite diagnosis may make doctors feel inadequate, and perhaps it is natural to counter this by giving the patient something definite, such as a prescription. Doctors may feel very uncomfortable doing nothing, because they think that the patient wants them to do something. In the past this has led to the widespread use of treatments thought to be placebos, such as 'tonics' or antibiotics for viral infections. If these remedies are prescribed with sufficient authority and confidence, the patient may well feel better, with the improvement attributable to the placebo effect. This course of action can be attractive, as the patient feels better and the doctor also feels better as she has responded to a request for help in a positive way. The downside lies in the deception to the patient and the fostering of expectations in patients for further prescriptions.

Is there any way of harnessing the placebo effect without deception or using prescriptions? According to one definition 'the placebo response is a change in the patient's health or bodily state that is attributable to the symbolic impact of medical treatment or the treatment setting' (Brody 2000, p.650). This indicates that the placebo effect may be achieved through the interaction between doctor and patient, rather than relying upon a prescription or other physical object. Brody suggests that developing the GP–patient relationship through strategies such as knowing and being interested in the patient, being caring, empathic, reliable, trustworthy and attentive to the patient's interests, and encouraging the patient to participate in decisions, will support the efficacy of the placebo effect. This may be a way of keeping the therapeutic power of the doctor–patient relationship without being paternalistic. Trust can play a significant role here: honesty about uncertainty may build trust and help to transfer the power of the placebo effect from the prescription to the doctor herself, thereby avoiding problems of deception. The GP can use existing trust within the relationship to 'ask for credit'; for example, to explain that even though she is not certain of a diagnosis, serious problems have been ruled out, and the problem will almost certainly get better on its own. This kind of approach may be as powerful as a physical placebo, especially if delivered with a positive attitude.

What is the medical good? The role of evidence-based medicine

If doctors are to act for the good of their patients, it is important that they know which treatments are effective and which are not. This is one of the main aims of evidence-based medicine (EBM), which attempts to ground healthcare in interventions that have been shown to be effective. At first glance, this aim fits in very well with ideas about acting in the patient's best interests, as it is surely in their interests to receive effective rather than ineffective or harmful treatments. Is using EBM a practical way of assisting GPs to act beneficently? There are some features about general practice that mean that using EBM to inform decision-making can be difficult, especially if GPs take an holistic approach to patient's interests (Rogers 2002; Slowther *et al.* 2004), and there are some features of EBM which raise doubts about its reliability.

First, much of the evidence for EBM comes from randomized controlled trials, in which the trial population is restricted to a relatively homogenous group with a single disease. In general practice, the population may be far more varied (with regard to age, gender or ethnicity) than the research population, so that it is not clear whether the findings are applicable. More significantly, co-morbidities are common in general practice, yet people with co-morbidities are excluded from most randomized controlled trials (Watt 2002).

Second, EBM reviews provide statistical estimates about the effectiveness of particular treatments in trials. This process necessarily reflects the existing research body, leading to questions about who develops and funds the research agenda, and who chooses which interventions to investigate. Over two-thirds of pharmaceutical research is funded by industry (Bekelman *et al.* 2003; House of Commons Health Committee 2005). This gives industry a powerful role in creating an evidence base to support pharmaceutical rather than any other kinds of intervention, especially the complex interventions that may be appropriate for general practice. This process leaves no room for input from patients as to the kind of interventions that they would prefer or find most acceptable.

As well as shaping the research agenda, industry exerts a significant influence over what is published in the literature (Smith 2005). Over half of the most cited trials published between 1994 and 2004 were funded solely by industry (Patsopoulos *et al.* 2006), indicating the influence of industry funding. In addition, there is growing evidence that the source of funding influences the results of the research, creating questions about the reliability of the results of industry funded research (Ridker and Torres 2006; Sismondo 2007).

Finally, and most importantly, evidence alone is insufficient to determine patient management. There are other important factors that feed into general practice decisions, including the preferences of the patient, the GP's knowledge of this particular patient or information about the local availability of services. Knowledge about effectiveness is rarely enough on its own to reach a conclusion, as we need information about the goals of the patient before it makes sense to ask whether a particular treatment is an effective way of reaching those goals. EBM can lead to an excessive focus on the scientific basis of medicine, which may be inappropriate for general practice, where personal and contextual features are an important part of practice (Slowther *et al.* 2004).

In practice, clinical guidelines are the working face of EBM. Evidence-based guidelines are developed using the principles of EBM, providing guidance for particular clinical scenarios. Many of these guidelines are quite paternalistic. Guidelines–for example, those produced by the UK National Institute for Clinical Excellence, the Australian National Institute for Clinical Studies or the Scottish Inter-collegiate Guidelines Network–tend to define a single management path without offering the opportunity for patients to choose amongst alternatives. There is a sort of shift here: instead of the GP being the medical expert, the guideline is now the expert who tells both the patient and the GP what to do. This may be seen as a new paternalism, with the relevant expertise now lying with the EBM guidelines and their authors, rather than the treating clinician. The pressure to follow the guidelines rather than tailor treatment to the individual patient may be exacerbated by financial or other incentives for GPs to follow EBM guidelines (Rogers 2002; Slowther *et al.* 2004).

This may seem to be a fairly gloomy account of EBM and its potential contribution to acting for the patient's good. However, the development of EBM has been accompanied by a growing interest in using evidence to assist patient decision-making, with evidence being synthesized into various decision aids. Reviews of patient decision aids indicate that they can have a number of beneficial effects for patients, including improved knowledge and participation in decision-making, and improved agreement between patients' values and the choices that they make (O'Connor *et al.* 2003).

In summary, EBM is one important source of information for GPs and, if there is relevant and credible data about the effectiveness of treatments, this should be used in patient care. GPs, however, describe various sources for their expertise, including professional experience, reading journals, personal experience, continuing medical education programmes and discussion with colleagues (Rogers 1999). The balance between EBM and these other sources of expertise is something to be weighed up for each patient.

The limits of beneficence

Acting in the patient's best interests is a moral imperative for doctors, but at times this imperative comes into conflict with other considerations. These kinds of conflicts may be difficult to identify, and can cause significant unease. In the following sections we discuss some examples of the limits of beneficence.

Patient-driven constraints

When consultations are patient-initiated, we trust that the patient is motivated by their health interests. By and large this is the case: patients come to see GPs because they have a health problem and GPs are able to use their skills in addressing the problem. Conflicts may arise when the patient's aims diverge from the GP's, away from the course of action that seems indicated by considerations of health.

Case 6.4

Mrs Duke is a patient in her late-60s, who is an infrequent attendee at the Gordon Road practice. One day she presented to Dr McFarlane with abdominal distension and anorexia. On examination, Dr McFarlane found a large mass and ascites. Dr McFarlane thought that the most likely diagnosis was ovarian cancer. She explained this to Mrs Duke and advised that some investigations would help to confirm the diagnosis and then it would be possible to work out what, if any, treatment would be recommended. Mrs Duke refused to have any investigations or to see a specialist for further assessment. She died at home several months later.

In this case, Mrs Duke came to see Dr McFarlane for a diagnosis, and then chose to decline further treatment, despite the explanations and encouragement of Dr McFarlane. In this kind of situation, the medical instinct and training is to investigate and treat the underlying pathology, in the hope that this process will lead to some good for the patient. When this offer of help is refused, this can be hard to accept. Why is this so hard? Partly perhaps because medicine just is a very practical occupation, geared towards doing something rather than nothing. Inactivity can feel like failure. A rejection of medical attention can feel like a personal rejection of the doctor herself, given the close links between professional skills and personal identity. A situation like this in which the harms to the patient are so grave, can severely test the limits of our commitment to patient self-determination. There is often the feeling that perhaps the patient did not understand about the diagnosis or likely consequences, or possibility for treatment, or perhaps the GP should have tried a bit harder to explain things. This is an important point: before accepting a refusal of treatment with potentially harmful consequences, we must ensure that the patient fully understands the implications of their decision.

How can we tell if a refusal is informed? The criteria for informed refusals are the same as for informed consent (see Chapter 8 for a full discussion of informed consent):

1. The patient must be competent to make the decision.

2. The doctor must provide enough information so that the patient can fully understand the nature and effects of the treatment that is recommended, and the likely consequences of refusing treatment.

3. The patient must make the decision voluntarily, without any coercion or manipulation from other people.

Why do patients like Mrs Duke refuse treatment? There is no single answer to this question, as people will refuse treatments for different reasons (Kleffens and Leeuwen 2005). However, in each situation where there is a risk of serious harm to the patient, it is part of good practice for the GP to ask about the patient's reasoning and try to understand why they are refusing treatment (Connelly 2000). This effort to understand on the part of the GP plays two ethical roles. First, listening to the patient demonstrates a commitment to care and trustworthiness, even though the doctor might prefer a different outcome. Second, by eliciting the patient's reasons for refusal, the GP can correct any misunderstandings and be satisfied that the refusal is fully informed.

If we consider the role of the patient in deciding her own good, and accept that medical care is only part of that good, refusals of treatment are a justifiable limit on beneficence. Beneficence requires that we do our best to offer medical care; patients, however, are not obliged to accept our offer. Imposing care upon people who do not want it is strongly paternalistic and violates patient autonomy. Chapter 8 explores patient autonomy more fully.

Complete refusals of medical care are relatively rare. More commonly, patients partially accept medical advice.

Case 6.5

Mr Jason Allen is a 29-year-old man with moderately severe asthma who smokes 10–15 cigarettes per day. He takes regular inhaled steroids and bronchodilators, but usually requires a short course of oral steroids for exacerbations of his asthma several times per year. His GP, Dr Carter, finds it very frustrating to see Mr Allen. He cannot understand why Mr Allen will not give up smoking.

From a medical point of view, Mr Allen's behaviour is unsatisfactory, as he will almost certainly see an improvement in his asthma if he gives up smoking.

There is a clear medical view about what is in this patient's best interests in relation to his health. However, Mr Allen does not follow medical advice and seems quite content to carry on smoking and to use oral steroids for his exacerbations.

What are the ethical considerations here? Dr Carter has a duty to act for the good of Mr Allen and to prevent harms, but achieving this good relies upon the patient changing his behaviour. Does Mr Allen have any obligation to follow medical advice? In general, medical ethicists have considered that patients always have the right to refuse treatment, and that there is no definite obligation to accept medical advice. There are also fairly universal legal prohibitions on treating patients against their will. However, part of being a trustworthy patient (as discussed in Chapter 3) is that the patient is genuinely seeking healthcare. In cases like that of Mr Allen, Dr Carter may find it helpful to clarify with Mr Allen what his aims are, and how these may be understood in the context of appearing to ignore medical advice. Despite the difficulty of working with patients who seem to be wilfully damaging their health, GPs are committed to providing healthcare and should not withhold services, even if they feel that the patient is compromising their medical care one way or another. It might be worth asking whether Dr Carter would feel differently if Mr Allen were an enthusiastic jogger and often presented to the surgery with injuries related to his jogging? The obligation remains to do the best medically for the patient, despite any feelings on the part of the GP of approval or disapproval about the patient's health-affecting actions.

Patients who attend frequently with illnesses that are exacerbated by their own behaviours raise questions about justice and resource allocation. If Mr Allen followed medical advice, this would decrease his need for medical services, reducing pressure on the system and leaving Dr Carter more time to see other patients. Do citizens within publicly funded healthcare systems have an obligation to limit their demands on the available resources? It seems reasonable to say that people have a duty not to use health services carelessly or casually, as by doing this they can divert attention away from more urgent cases; for example, calling an ambulance for a sprained wrist or calling for a home visit for a repeat prescription (Draper and Sorrell 2002). But who should be the judge of careful use? This is where the difficulties start, as fear and lack of knowledge can be potent triggers for actions that might seem unwarranted from a medical perspective. The nature of general practice offers the opportunity for GPs to discuss with patients the best way to use the healthcare that they offer (see Chapter 7 for a full discussion of justice and resource allocation).

Practitioner-driven constraints and medical responsibility

Are there any limits to the extent of GPs' commitment to act for their patients' good? We can break down the duty of beneficence into four parts:

1. One ought not to inflict evil or harm.

2. One ought to prevent evil or harm.

3. One ought to remove evil.

4. One ought to do or promote good (Frankena 1973, p.47).

Following this account, GPs are more obliged to prevent or remove harms than to do good, and this ties in with our intuitions and some empirical observations (Rogers 1999). Healthcare does seem to have adopted this hierarchy, with its greater obligation to act to prevent harms than to promote good–just think of the way that medical budgets are split between acute and preventive services. But, what of the limits to doing or promoting good? Does this create a potentially limitless demand to perform supererogatory actions on behalf of patients? This issue is particularly challenging in general practice, where there is less distinction between the patient's health interests and their overall interests, compared with secondary or tertiary care. It may be difficult to define clear limits to medical responsibility. For almost every consultation it is possible to think of some extra effort or action that could have benefited the patient; these feelings are compounded by the time pressures operating in much of general practice. For example, should Dr Singh have offered to negotiate with Barry Black's boss in Case 6.2, or even helped him with some financial support, as both of these actions may improve Barry's medical outcome? Most people would answer 'No' to these suggestions, as they are outside the boundaries of medical care; but it is possible to think of cases–for example, advocating for a patient to receive supported housing–where the limits are not so clear.

Conflict may occur between GPs and patients if patients request medical services that GPs consider unnecessary. For example, guidelines and reviews on the management of low back pain advise that plain lumbar X-rays should not be performed routinely. Not only are they unlikely to help diagnostically, there are the potential harms of incidental findings and exposure to irradiation. From a medical perspective, these are quite powerful reasons to refuse requests for an X-ray. But what of the patient who, for whatever reason, is not reassured by this line of reasoning? Perhaps they know someone who was also refused an X-ray for back pain who turned out to have cancer, perhaps it is just not possible for that person to accept a diagnosis of soft tissue strain unless they have seen for themselves that there is nothing wrong with their bones. There is no single way to resolve problems of this kind that require balancing up the various factors case by case. On the one hand, there are pressures to do with practising scientific medicine, not wasting resources and adhering to standards of care, but on the other hand, refusing a request may compromise the therapeutic relationship with the patient and fail to recognize important facts about that particular patient.

External constraints

Acting in the patient's best interests can be constrained by external circumstances, such as lack of resources to follow medically-indicated courses of actions or requirements to adhere to mandated standards of care dictated by approved guidelines. Most publicly funded health systems face shortages in some areas. In the National Health Service in the UK, for example, patients are faced with waiting lists for investigations, referrals and treatments, whilst in other countries there may be a limited set of options available for the GP to access for their patients. At times GPs may find themselves forced to choose between an externally mandated standard of care and what they feel to be in the best interests of this particular patient, based upon their personal knowledge and communication with the patient. This problem is most acute when care is audited according to external standards, with implications for practice accreditation and/or financing.

In some ways, external constraints do not cause the same ethical distress as challenges related to patient choices. This might be because GPs do not feel responsible for the short-comings of state healthcare systems in the way that they might feel responsible for some of the actions of their patients. Once a course of action has been determined and the patient is waiting for a service, pressure eases on the GP and patients do not usually hold GPs responsible for any failings of the wider healthcare service.

However, external constraints do raise ethical issues, especially when access to specialists through the state-funded system may take months, whilst private appointments can be obtained at very short notice; as, for example, is the case in Australia. Private access to secondary and tertiary services creates a double standard of healthcare, with those who can afford to receiving a much swifter service. If these patients are then slotted into public operating lists, ahead of people waiting for public out-patients' appointments, the injustice is compounded.

Preventive healthcare

One area of healthcare that raises specific questions about beneficence is preventive care. Preventive activities including screening, vaccination and health promotion are now within the mainstream business of general practice, reflecting international trends towards prevention. It is usually taken for granted that prevention is better than cure. In relation to ethics, the most significant reason why prevention is better than cure is that prevention avoids the harms of disease, making it part of the duty of beneficence, which includes preventing harms and promoting goods such as good health. If we accept that health is valuable and that individuals are harmed by ill health, then we have an ethical reason to try to prevent ill health. Preventive healthcare has the potential to prevent some diseases or to achieve better treatment outcomes through earlier identification of diseases than would otherwise occur. There are also economic reasons why prevention may be better than cure, as preventing disease may be cheaper than treating it, although the economic arguments are not infallible.

Both the ethical and the medical views about prevention direct us towards performing at least some preventive activities; however, there are some ethical concerns (see Box 6.3).

Box 6.3 Ethical issues raised by preventive care

Balancing beneficence and autonomy:

- What pressures are there to ensure patient compliance?
- Has the patient given informed consent?
- Is there an acceptable and effective treatment?
- Is there a duty to avoid harming others?

Preventing harms:

- What is the balance of benefits over harms, short and long term?
- How do the harms and benefits affect individuals versus populations?
- Do the preventive activities lead to medicalization and the potential for victim blaming?

Justice:

- Who receives the preventive care and what is the impact upon inequalities in health?
- How are resources allocated between prevention and treatment?

Balancing beneficence and autonomy

Preventive care highlights the tensions that may occur between balancing the two ethical duties of beneficence and respect for autonomy. Preventive care is based upon acting for the good of the person receiving the care, in terms of avoiding or minimizing harms. This is a strong moral foundation, but can be compromised if there are undue pressures to make sure that patients comply with preventive care. Pressures may come from external sources; for example, government targets for immunizations or cervical cancer screening that link financial rewards to rates of immunization or screening. This creates a potential conflict of interests for the GP. To act in the best interests of the patient requires that the GP explain the preventive activity and seek informed consent, with the final decision left up to the patient. However, if the patient refuses, this may affect the GP's income. Patients who realize that GPs have a financial interest in achieving preventive care targets may feel that they are coerced; for example, by receiving multiple and unsolicited reminders to attend for cervical cancer screening. (See also Chapter 12 on conflicts of interest.)

Many preventive activities are routine, such as recording risk factors or measuring blood pressure. We often take consent for granted in these cases, but for some preventive activities, more formal informed consent is critical. This can be difficult, especially when the information is hard to assemble or is equivocal. For some screening activities, such as cervical cancer screening, there have been no formal trials to prove effectiveness; for other forms of screening, such as for prostate cancer, the evidence of benefit in terms of reduced mortality is equivocal; and, for colorectal cancer screening, there may be a lack of agreement as to the best method of screening due to variations in sensitivity, specificity, cost and safety of the different methods (Jatoi and Anderson 2005).

Beneficence requires that the actions taken for the patient's good do actually benefit the person. Therefore it is important to be sure that screening for early detection of a disease will actually lead to a benefit to the patient from the early detection. In most cases, this means that there must be an effective, acceptable and accessible intervention (Juth and Munthe 2007).

The threats posed by infectious diseases raise interesting questions about the scope of the obligation that patients (as citizens) might have to prevent illness in others. At the least onerous level, there is a duty to avoid unnecessary contact with others whilst suffering from an infectious disease, such as influenza or gastroenteritis, or to avoid spreading sexually transmitted infections. But what are the limits? Do people have an obligation to avoid all contact with others during the flu season to avoid transmission or to get vaccinated in order to avoid accidental infection and transmission? (Verweij 2007). There is an emerging body of literature on the ethics of infectious diseases that engages with these issues (Selgelid *et al.* 2006).

Preventing harms

Part of the ethical complexity of preventive care and screening lies in trying to balance an abstract and often quite small risk for a patient against the possible harms from the intervention. For example, lowering cholesterol levels across the population will lead to a measurable and significant decrease in heart disease; but for any one individual, the decrease in risk may be negligible. This is the prevention paradox, first described by Rose: actions to improve health on the part of individuals often show a benefit at the population level but not for that particular individual (Rose 1985). When the preventive action involves making changes that are quite intrusive into the life of the patient, such as major dietary changes, we need to be certain that the benefits are worth the effort for the patient. Technical information can help to inform decisions, such as the rates of false-positives and negatives, the predictive value of the test, and the possible consequences of a false positive. What happens to a person with a positive test, in terms of further investigations, and how should we measure the fear and anxiety felt, for example, by a person with a positive faecal occult blood test who is waiting for further investigations?

A second potential harm with preventive healthcare is known as medicalization. This refers to the phenomenon of currently healthy people adjusting the way that they live in response to medical information or advice; for example, taking more exercise, eating different foods, undergoing screening examinations and so forth. The ethical problems associated with medicalization are threefold: increased levels of worry and concern about one's health; potential victim-blaming for those who appear not to take responsibility for their health; and a focus on health as an unduly prominent value in life (Verweij 2007).

The onus for avoiding harms is higher for preventive healthcare than for ordinary care sought by the patient. Preventive activities are usually instigated by the healthcare practitioner or other third party, rather than coming at the patient's own request, which changes the potential balance of benefits and harms. If the patient voluntarily seeks healthcare in response to symptoms or concerns, there is an existing harm (the problem for which they are seeking care) that can be weighed up against any possible harms and benefits from investigations and treatment. In preventive healthcare, there is no existing harm: the patient is healthy, not actively seeking treatment and the harm to be avoided through the preventive activity is only potential. Given these conditions, the safety and efficacy of preventive healthcare are paramount.

Justice: what is the impact upon inequalities in health?

One of the major ethical issues raised by preventive care and health promotion is that these activities are more likely to taken up by people living in more well-off socio-economic circumstances than by people living in more deprived circumstances (Acheson 1998). This means that, although the health of some (well-off) groups may be improved, the benefits are not always spread evenly and there can be a widening of the existing health gap. In addition, the focus upon the individual and their role in being healthy takes no account of the structural features of societies that lead to ill health. Preventive healthcare programmes aimed at individuals are unlikely to exert a major impact upon population health or to reduce the health gap, unless accompanied by programmes to address the more deeply rooted causes of ill health such as discrimination, financial hardship, lack of education and so forth.

Finally, there is the issue of resource allocation. How much should governments spend upon preventive versus acute healthcare services; and for GPs, how much time should they allocate to prevention given the inevitable pressures on the consultation? There is an ever increasing number of preventive activities, currently estimated to be up to 25 separate preventive interventions for a typical general practice patient (Russell 2005). Preventive healthcare can offer undoubted benefits, especially at a population level, but at times the current needs of the patient override these.

Conclusion

Acting for the good of patients is one of the fundamental ethical requirements of medical practice. In this chapter we have explored some of the complexities that may arise when GPs try to act for the good of their patients, and the relationship between beneficence and paternalism. Sometimes patients themselves may act in ways that hinder their medical interests, and sometimes external circumstances can lead to less than optimal care. Health prevention activities raise their own challenges, as the expected benefits may be difficult to predict with accuracy, informed choices of patients may be compromised and there are risks of medicalization. Finally, we have briefly raised the issue of justice; this is explored fully in the next chapter.

References

Acheson D (1998). *Independent inquiry into inequalities in health*. Stationery Office, London.

Bekelman JE, Li Y and Gross CP (2003). Scope and impact of financial conflicts of interest in biomedical research: a systematic review. *Journal of the American Medical Association* **289**, 454–465.

Brody H (2000). The placebo response: recent research and the implications for family medicine. *Journal of Family Practice* **49**, 649–654.

Childress JF (2007). Paternalism in healthcare and health policy. In Ashcroft RE, Dawson R, Draper H and McMillan JR (ed.) *Principles of heath care ethics* (2nd edn). John Willey & Sons Ltd, Chichester, England, 223–229.

Christie R and Hoffmaster B (1986). *Ethical issues in family medicine.* Oxford University Press, New York.

Connelly J (2000). Refusal of treatment. In Sugarman J (ed.) *Ethics in primary care.* McGraw-Hill Health Professions Division, New York.

Downie R and Calman K (1994). *Healthy respect: ethics in healthcare* (2nd edn). Oxford Medical Publications, Oxford.

Draper H and Sorrell T (2002). Patients' responsibilities in medical ethics. *Bioethics* **16**, 335–352.

General Medical Council (2006). *Good medical practice* (paragraphs 72c and 74). Available from http://www.gmc-uk.org/guidance/good_medical_practice/index.asp (accessed 23 April 2008).

Frankena W (1973). *Ethics* (2nd edn). Prentice Hall Inc, New Jersey.

Häyry H (1998) Paternalism. In Chadwick R (ed.) *Encyclopedia of applied ethics*, Academic Press, San Diego, vol. 3, 449–457.

House of Commons Health Committee (2005). *The influence of the pharmaceutical industry.* Available from http://www.lindalliance.org/pdfs/HofCHealthCommittee.pdf (accessed 23 April 2008).

Jatoi I and Anderson WF (2005). Cancer screening. *Current Problems in Surgery* **42**, 620–682.

Juth N and Munthe C (2007). Screening and ethical aspects. In Ashcroft RE, Dawson R, Draper H, McMillan JR (ed.) *Principles of heath care ethics* (2nd edn) John Willey & Sons Ltd, Chichester, England, 607–615.

Katz J (1984). *The silent world of doctor and patient.* Free Press, New York.

Kleffens TV and Leeuwen EV (2005). Physicians' evaluations of patients' decisions to refuse oncolgical treatment. *Journal of Medical Ethics* **31**, 131–136.

Little P, Everitt H, Williamson I, Warner G, Moore M, Gould C, Ferrier K and Payne S (2001). Observational study of the effect of patient centredness and positive approach on outcomes of general practice consultations. *British Medical Journal* **323**, 908–911.

O'Connor AM, Stacey D, Entwistle V, Llewellyn-Thomas H, Rovner D, Holmes-Rovner M, Tait V, Tetroe J, Fiset V, Barry M and Jones J (2003). Decisions aids for people facing health treatment of screening decisions. *Cochrane Database of Systematic Reviews* (2):CD001431.

Patsopoulos NA, Analatos AA and Ioannidis JPA (2006). Origin and finding of the most frequently cited papers in medicine: database and analysis. *British Medical Journal* **332**, 1061–1064.

Ridker PM and Torres J (2006). Reported outcomes in major cardiovascular clinical trials funded by for-profit and not-for-profit organizations: 2000–2005. *Journal of the American Medical Association* **295**, 2270–2274.

Rogers WA (1999). Beneficence in general practice: an empirical investigation. *Journal of Medical Ethics* **25**(5), 388–393.

Rogers WA (2002). Are guidelines ethical? Some considerations for general practice. *British Journal of General Practice* **52**, 663–669.

Rose G (1985). Sick individuals and sick populations. *International Journal of Epidemiology* **14**, 32–38.

Russel GM (2005). Is prevention unbalancing general practice? *Medical Journal Australia* **183**, 104–105.

Savage R and Armstrong D (1990). Effect of a general practitioner's consulting style on patients' satisfaction: a controlled study. *British Medical Journal* **301**, 968–970.

Selgelid M, Battin M and Smith CB (2006). *Ethics and infectious disease.* Blackwell Publishing, Oxford, UK.

Sherwin S (1992). *No longer patient.* Temple University Press, Philadelphia.

Sismondo S (2007). Ghost management: How much of the medical literature is shaped behind the scenes by the pharmaceutical industry? *PLoS Medicine* **4**(9): e286.

Slowther A, Ford S and Schofield T (2004). Ethics of evidence based medicine in the primary care setting. *Journal of Medical Ethics* **30**, 151–156.

Smith R (2005). Medical journals are an extension of the marketing arm of pharmaceutical companies. *PLoS Medicine* **2**(5), e138.

Thomas K (1987). General practice consultations: is there any point in being positive? *British Medical Journal* **294**, 1200–1202.

Verweij M (2007). Preventing disease. In Ashcroft RE, Dawson R, Draper H and McMillan JR (ed.) *Principles of heath care ethics* (2nd edn). John Willey & Sons Ltd, Chichester, England, 557–562.

Watt G (2002). The inverse care law today. *Lancet* **360**, 252–254.

Wikipedia (2008). Hippocratic oath. http://en.wikipedia.org/wiki/Hippocratic__Oath (accessed 19 August 2008).

Chapter 7

Justice and resource allocation in general practice

Case 7.1

Dr Martin Schroeder occasionally works in the Hackney Road Practice in inner city London. Jennifer is Dr Schroeder's sixth appointment this morning. He has only met Jennifer once before, but he can tell immediately that Jennifer seems tired and flat. Yet, Jennifer's reasons for presenting seem very minor. She's worried that a fall 3 months ago on the steps outside her house may be the reason she cannot conceive. She already has two children, each conceived after a year of trying. She and her partner have been trying for a pregnancy for 6 months now. After examining her, and finding no evidence of any effects of the fall, Dr Schroeder tries to reassure Jennifer that a minor fall is unlikely to stop her conceiving. He suggests that Jennifer return at the end of the year if she is still not pregnant and her regular doctor can begin some investigations then. On the tip of Dr Schroeder's tongue are the words, 'You seem very down in the dumps, Jennifer. Is anything else troubling you?' but, Dr Schroeder is already running 30 minutes late, and he has a busy clinic still ahead of him. He tells himself: 'Maybe I'm not being fair to her, but if I get further behind now, I'll never catch up. And, she'll come back again if there's really something wrong.'

Case 7.2

Dr Carter scans the day's appointments. He notices Mr Servante has another appointment for 10.00 a.m. and his heart sinks. Mr Servante's multiple problems (headaches, irritable bowel syndrome, joint pains, tiredness) always have to be dealt with immediately. He is usually worried that Dr Carter is hiding something from him and so he refuses to leave until Dr Carter has slowly and carefully explained every detail. Dr Carter expects to be running at least one hour late by the time Mr Servante leaves. 'It's not fair', he thinks to himself. 'Every other patient I see today suffers because of him.'

Case 7.3

Dr Day has known Simone since she was 1-year-old, when he first joined the practice. Now Simone is 25, a secretary in the district council office, about half an hour's drive away. She is an attractive woman but, from her point of view, she has one major problem: her nose. Simone's nose is large and she believes it completely disfigures her face. She is convinced that the reason she can not attract and keep a boyfriend is because no man will look twice at someone with a nose her size.

Since Simone first raised this issue with him about five years ago Dr Day has come to understand that, for whatever reason, Simone's nose really does impact significantly on her life. She is often depressed and she presents regularly with ill-defined aches and pains that never really seem to resolve. He has facilitated access to counselling through the regional health service but this has not really helped. In fact, the mental health nurse implied that cosmetic surgery might indeed be a good solution for Simone's problems. At her urging, Dr Day has tried to get Simone in to see a plastic surgeon to have her assessed. But here's the problem: Australia's public hospitals do not provide cosmetic surgery free of charge except for a small number of very limited conditions, so Simone will not be able to have cosmetic surgery as a public patient.

Today Simone is sitting in front of Dr Day in tears. He has just told her that, if she wants her nose fixed, she will need to be treated in the private sector. Both of them know this is unrealistic, for Simone's means are modest and she has no private health insurance. 'It's just not fair', she sobs, 'Isn't there anything we can do about it?'

This chapter is about allocating resources fairly in a general practice setting. Our examples set the scene. Although they are very different, reflecting both differences in funding arrangements for health services between countries and different clinical scenarios, in each case people are concerned with the same problem: 'It's not fair'. When we talk about things as being fair or unfair, just or unjust, what do we mean? And how can we decide what the 'fair' or 'just' thing might be?

Problems such as these can pose troubling dilemmas for many doctors. Resolution of resource allocation dilemmas can be assisted by a thoughtful consideration of the ways in which decisions are being made, and an analysis of the criteria for a just distribution. This chapter deals with these issues. We begin with a definition of resource allocation and a general discussion of the many ways in which resources are shared out in various health systems. This is followed by a philosophical discussion of theories and principles of justice, focusing on four criteria for the allocation of healthcare resources: allocation according to need; capacity to benefit; merit; and rights.

What is resource allocation and why does it matter?

Resource allocation involves the distribution of goods and services to people, programmes or projects. In healthcare, resource allocation takes place at a number of levels. At the level of *macroallocation*, it concerns decisions, often made by government or health officials, about which programmes will be supported and to what degree. Such decisions are not limited to healthcare; they also concern how much to allocate to other social goods, such as housing, education and transport. Programmes outside the 'health budget' will often have impacts on health; for example, transport policy can impact on health through decisions about road upgrades, the presence of speed cameras or the provision of bicycle lanes.

Within the health budget, decisions need to be made about how to allocate the available monies. So, for example, governments must make decisions about the degree of emphasis they place on health promotion and preventive services for children, as opposed to, say, care and treatment services for children who have life-threatening illnesses.

At the level of *mesoallocation,* resource allocation decisions are made within institutions. How will the local hospital distribute its budget between the various services it provides? Should the regional health service support an intensive visiting programme for new mothers and their babies? On a smaller scale, general practitioners also make mesoallocation decisions; for example, when the topic of the practice meeting turns to the distribution of the practice budget. Do we employ a part-time mental health nurse, or would it be better to increase the hours for the practice accountant?

Microallocation decisions relate to individual patients. In general practice, problems of microallocation occur, for instance, when a GP has to decide if she will make an important house call first or see that patient who has been in the waiting room for the last hour. Both Dr Schroeder and Dr Carter are making micro-allocation decisions when they decide either to cut short a potentially lengthy consultation or to allow a consultation to run on.

What all these situations have in common is that there is not enough money, time, staff, machines or other resources available to do everything for every patient. Butler puts the problem in this way:

> Whether care is organized as a tax-funded services that is free at the point of use or as a commercial enterprise for which people pay directly or through insurance, it is

simply not possible to offer the full spectrum of clinical possibilities to every patient at every stage of life. The cost would be unsustainable, whether it fell on citizens as tax-payers or on patients as fee-payers.

(Butler 1999, p.6).

Scarcity is thus an inevitable characteristic of any health system.

Although a GP's prime responsibility is to the individual patient, there are at least two reasons why GPs can not avoid resource allocation issues completely. First, scarcity is a characteristic of many of the services GPs themselves provide. As we have seen above, it is often the GPs' *time* that is the scarce resource. In addition, general practitioners have a crucial role to play in resource allocation decisions beyond their own practices because they are often 'gatekeepers' to other services offered within the healthcare system. In many countries GPs stand at the gate to other health services, deciding who should be let through. In addition, they use their professional judgement to decide which treatments and services are warranted for which patients. Even in health systems that do not accord the GP a gatekeeper role, they still play an important role in advising and advocating for patients. When GPs use both their own resources and those they gate-keep wastefully, less resources are available for their patients and for those of other doctors.

How are resources allocated in healthcare systems?

Before we turn to a discussion of principles and theories of justice, it is worth noting the range of rationing options that are used on a daily basis. Butler provides a list of the strategies that are actually used within the National Health Service in the United Kingdom. Although this list was written with one country in mind, the same strategies are used in countries around the world.

First, Butler suggests that one way governments can address the problem of rationing health services and treatment is by being explicit about their healthcare priorities. This approach has been used in Britain for a long time; for example, from the NHS's stated priority for the elderly and the mentally ill in the 1970s, through to setting targets for morbidity and mortality in specific disease areas in the 1990s. In a similar way, the Dutch Government Committee on Choices in Healthcare in 1991 advised that mandatory health insurance schemes should address four questions in deciding on the content of a basic package of healthcare services: is the service necessary for an individual to participate in social and public life?; is it effective?; is it efficient?; and can it be left to individual responsibility (van de Ven 1995)? Whether these priority setting approaches work is another matter; there is some evidence to suggest that, despite blueprints and guidelines from government to address priorities explicitly, resources do not necessarily shift from areas of lower priority to areas of higher priority.

Box 7.1 The variety of rationing approaches

Articulating explicit priorities for health care.

Removing services from the menu of those on offer.

Relying on the courts.

Reducing the demand for care by discouraging people from entering the system.

Reducing the demand for care by slowing people's progress through the system.

Enhancing the efficiency and effectiveness of care.

Re-focusing attention towards prevention.

Devolving rationing responsibility to clinicians.

(Adapted from Butler 1999, pp.16–36.)

A second way in which the rationing problem can be addressed is to remove some services completely and to shift the resources that would be allocated to these services to others. For example, in the United Kingdom local health authorities do make decisions to drop certain treatments off the list of services that they make available to patients in their regions; the most common ones have been 'reversal of female sterilization, in vitro fertilization, sex change operations, breast augmentation, rhinoplasty, the reversal of male vasectomy, the removal of tattoos, and cosmetic surgery for varicose veins' (Butler 1999, p.21). In the Netherlands, a range of services were removed from the basic health service package during the 1990s; these included medically unnecessary cosmetic surgery, homeopathic remedies, spectacles and lenses, dental services for adults, long term physiotherapy and a number of ineffective drugs (van der Grinten and Kasdorp 1999).

When governments and health authorities exclude treatments from their list of services, they appear to make decisions either because there is relevant scientific evidence available (for example, excluding ear grommets and ineffective drugs) or because it seems that the desired treatment or service is a matter of private preference rather than health need (for example, cosmetic surgery). Often there is little debate about these issues and the reasons that underpin them in the public sphere.

A third way in which rationing decisions occur is through the courts. Historically, in most countries the courts have tended to avoid making legal judgments in this arena, preferring to regard such decisions as the proper responsibility of government, health authorities and clinicians. In recent years, however, the courts have begun to scrutinize resource allocation decisions more carefully, to demand explanations for those decisions and, occasionally, to return decisions to health authorities and governments for reconsideration (Newdick 2004).

The strategies considered so far have focused on the supply side of the rationing problem. Other alternatives open to those who need to ration health services alter the demand for services. Butler suggests that we can influence demand for healthcare in two ways: we can try to discourage patients from entering the healthcare system (primary inhibitors) and we can slow down patients' progress once they are in the system (secondary inhibitors).

In countries in which GPs function as gatekeepers, primary inhibitors work principally through GPs and their practices. Examples of primary inhibitors are education campaigns for patients (for example, on sensible use of your GP), reception practices (answering services, triaging by reception staff, etc.) and appointment systems (which create a delay between a patient's intention to seek treatment and the service itself so that some people drop out in this period).

Once in the system, secondary inhibitors function to control demand. Delay in access to out-patient appointments or admission as in-patients is a well-known phenomenon to any GP. Dilution makes the services available but spreads it so thinly that each person gets a less than desirable service (Parker 1975). For example, fertility treatment may be restricted to one or two cycles. Another strategy in this stable is to dilute the expertise of staff, by employing more junior staff, or differently and less qualified staff, to deliver the service.

The sixth strategy used to ration services is to try to enhance the efficiency and effectiveness of the system. 'Efficiency... is about maximizing the quantity and quality of what is achieved from a given quantum of resource' (Butler 1999, p.31). Effectiveness, on the other hand, is not related to cost, but rather to how well a treatment works, usually when compared against other treatments. The rise of evidence-based medicine and its more applied counterpart, health technology assessment, are direct results of efforts to attend to both the efficiency and effectiveness of particular treatments. For example, in Australia the Medical Services Advisory Committee advises the Minister for Health and Ageing on the strength of evidence available on new and existing medical technologies and procedures in terms of their safety, effectiveness and cost-effectiveness. This advice assists the Australian Government in making decisions about which medical services should attract funding under the national health insurance scheme (Medical Services Advisory Committee 2008). Evidence-based medicine and health technology assessment do not, however, necessarily reduce the healthcare budget. For example, if we find a treatment to be effective, the pressure for it to be available to all will be considerable, regardless of the availability of resources to fund it.

A seventh way to manage the rationing problem is to re-focus healthcare, so that problems are prevented before they arise. We have discussed this issue in Chapter 6. Ethically, the arguments for and against prevention are complex, as prevention can often mean more paternalism on the part of government or doctors.

The final strategy that Butler notes is to devolve allocation decisions to clinicians. On a daily basis, GPs make many decisions about the allocation of resources (Butler 1999, p.35):

> It is as though there exists an unspoken social contract: 'society' has entrusted to the clinicians the responsibility for taking the ultimate decisions about the allocation of scarce resources, and in return 'society' has absolved the clinicians from explicit democratic accountability for their stewardship of that responsibility.

Mostly, such decisions happen with little awareness amongst the public more generally, although occasionally the popular press brings the attention of the general community to specific decisions.

Listing the range of ways in which rationing occurs is one thing; deciding whether such approaches are fair and morally acceptable is a different task altogether. Clearly, not all of these approaches to resource allocation are of equal moral worth, and the breadth and variety of strategies only reinforce the need for a rational and sound basis for distributing scarce healthcare resources. The rest of this chapter draws on principles and theories of justice to help us analyse different ways to allocate resources.

How can we allocate resources fairly?

Theories and principles of justice

At its most simple, justice is done when each person gets his or her due. This suggests that people who are equal with respect to their 'dues' ought to get the same amount. Indeed, all theories of justice, from Aristotle onwards, have had as a minimum formal requirement that equals shall be treated equally and unequals unequally. This is a 'formal' principle of justice, because it provides no detail about the circumstances under which equals should be treated equally and because it does not tell us whether two or more people are in fact equal.

Box 7.2 Formal principle of justice

The formal principle of justice states that equals shall be treated equally and unequals unequally.

Fleshing out the formal principle of justice is the chief issue in debates about distributive justice. Just what criteria can we use to decide whether people are equal or unequal? What is it about Mr Servante that makes Dr Carter thinks it unfair that he take up more surgery time than other patients? Should Simone be regarded as equal to other patients who have different treatment needs or wishes?

We need a way to give content to this formal principle of justice. There are really two routes we can take. The first route focuses on processes or procedures that we may use to allocate resources–this leads us to considerations of *procedural justice*. The second route concerns the characteristics of individuals or groups to whom resources may go and the outcomes resulting from that distribution. This route leads to the identification of *material principles of justice*.

Procedural justice

Procedural justice approaches the problem of fairness by suggesting that we can arrive at fair or just outcomes if the procedures that we use to allocate our resources are fair. One famous example of procedural justice is John Rawls' 'veil of ignorance' (Rawls 1972). Rawls asks us to imagine that we are in the hypothetical situation of deciding how to allocate a range of primary social goods (such as education and healthcare) in a society. He gives us total knowledge of the society that we are making decisions for, *but* we have absolutely no knowledge of what our personal position will be in that society. Behind this 'veil of ignorance', Rawls suggests that reasonable decision-makers will be able to allocate resources in a fair way.

A recent attempt to devise fair processes for the allocation of healthcare resources has come from the work of Daniels and Sabin (Daniels and Sabin 1997; Daniels 2000). In their 'accountability for reasonableness' approach, a fair allocation process must meet four conditions. First, the decision, and its rationale, must be publicly accessible to those it is going to affect. Second, the rationale for the decision should provide 'a *reasonable* construal of... how the organization (or society) should provide 'value for money' in meeting the varied health needs of a defined population in reasonable resource constraints' (Daniels and Sabin 1997, p.329). 'Reasonable' here is defined in terms of reasons that people who are being fair-minded can agree on as relevant to the situation. Daniels and Sabin's third condition is that there must be avenues for appeal and review of decisions, so that good arguments to modify decisions can be articulated, considered and fed back to help revise policy. Finally, a fair allocation process needs to have a mechanism, either voluntary or public, to enforce the first three conditions.

Generally, fair procedures in healthcare will not guarantee fair outcomes, but they will help. At a broad societal level, for example, citizens' referenda and community consultations have been used occasionally to decide which services will be provided with a geographic region. At more local levels, fair procedures can contribute significantly to fair outcomes. For example, the ways in which research ethics committees make decisions about which research will be allowed to proceed and which will not are significantly enhanced when the committee's activities are demonstrably impartial, transparent to interested parties and clear.

Material principles of justice

Philosophers label the ways that we give content to our formal principle of justice *material principles* of justice. These principles provide criteria that we can use to determine who should be entitled to receive the resources that are available. In a sense, they give us a range of standards that we may use to measure equality (or inequality) amongst people.

Different scholars offer different alternatives for material principles of justice. In this chapter, we will consider

- allocation of health resources according to need;
- allocation of health resources according to capacity to benefit;
- allocation of health resources according to merit; and
- allocation of health resources according to rights.

Obviously, the corollary of these statements is that people who have different needs or capacity to benefit or merit or rights should be treated differently. In the following section we examine each of these alternatives and to explore their strengths and weaknesses.

Choosing between people on the basis of need

The first way in which we can choose between people when allocating health resources is to allocate according to need. It seems obvious that people with equal need should have equal access to resources. Indeed, treatment on the basis of clinical need is often presented as the core characteristic of a health system (Butler 1999; van der Grinten and Kasdorp 1999). Allocating according to clinical need, such that people who are sick get treated and the sickest get treated first, has always been a guiding principle for doctors.

Yet, beneath this apparent simplicity lies a myriad of problems. 'Need' as a concept is hard to grasp firmly, in part because 'need' and 'want' are not always distinct. There are circumstances in which the two are clearly differentiated; for example, a patient's need for surgery to treat acute appendicitis is of a rather different order to his desire to be in a private room during his hospital stay. But there are other circumstances in which need and want are not so easy to distinguish. Cosmetic surgery, such as that desired by Simone, raises particularly sharply the confusion between needs and wants. When does a disfiguring nose become so significant that the desire to have a smaller nose become a legitimate health need? Dr Carter may also be thinking about the relationship between needs and desires when he grumbles about Mr Servante's lengthy consultations. From Dr Carter's point of view, Mr Servante may have a great desire for reassurance, but his actual need for treatment is fairly minor and probably less than other patients in the waiting room. If Dr Carter could organize his clinic so that he is treating according to need, Mr Servante would receive less time and other patients more.

The example of Dr Carter and Mr Servante raises a second problem for needs-based resource allocation. Just who should decide which needs are legitimate? This issue can be addressed to some extent by distinguishing between subjective and objective needs. Subjective needs are the needs that people define themselves as having. Objective needs are defined by someone else, often specific categories of people who have the authority to make judgements about the severity of need. In our society, it is often doctors who make decisions about whether a patient's need is objectively real or not. They may be helped (or hindered) in this task by professional guidelines or government policies that delineate the clinical indications for particular treatments; for example, GPs may be permitted to prescribe expensive drugs for only some conditions or for conditions that present in particular ways.

We might think that using a subjective needs-based criterion for the allocation of health resources would always result in patients wanting more than the GP might think reasonable and, conversely, that if we leave the judgment of need up to GPs, they will always deliver less than patients want. Certainly, this is what would seem to be happening in Mr Servante's case. However, Dr Schroeder's interaction with Jennifer casts this issue in a different light. Here, it is Dr Schroeder who is second-guessing an unacknowledged need in Jennifer. Dr Schroeder is using a rationing schema here that, at least partly, allocates GP time according to need only when the patient explicitly acknowledges her need. In daily practice, much of the resource allocating that GPs do is probably of this nature; it is a see-saw between patient-led identification of need and GP-led response to acknowledged need.

Even if doctor and patient can agree on the severity of the need, there are other problems for needs-based resource allocation. What are we to make of the fact that a significant proportion of the conditions GPs see just improve of their own accord over time? We might argue that these conditions could hardly be said to 'need' treatment at all. In these circumstances, should patients with these conditions be seen in GP surgeries at all? Or, would it be fairer to those patients with critical needs if minor self-limiting illnesses were assessed in other settings?

The final problem for needs-based allocation schemas is one that is noted by Butler (1999, pp.128–133). 'Needs' are not things that can exist outside of the resources that are available to meet them. Butler describes the case of an elderly woman with poor bladder control who is unable, because of arthritis, to get to the toilet quickly. She needs incontinence pads, but there is a local health authority policy that provides pads free of charge only to people with 'very debilitating illnesses' or as a complication of surgery. As this woman falls into neither of these categories, and because she is poor, she is often wet and has skin sores. In this situation, her need is for district nursing care for her skin sores. However, she would be better served if her need for incontinence pads, or for the money to buy them, could be met.

Sometime needs for healthcare arise out of situations that really demand other sorts of responses. For example, depression in a young, unemployed male might be better dealt with by finding him a job than by prescribing antidepressants. If the 'real' need can not be met by the health system, should the health system meet the 'substitute' need at all? Some of the underlying causes of ill-health lie in domains that GPs and other health professionals can influence very little (for example, poor housing). Here GPs are reduced to dealing with the consequences rather than the causes of ill health. How do we decide which services are legitimately the responsibility of a health system and which services fall outside its reach?

All of this suggests that need is not an all or nothing phenomenon–it is, as Butler suggests, an 'elastic' notion, that expands and contracts according to the social and economic environment. So, to allocate health services according to need is not at all straightforward.

So far, in talking about health needs we have focused on deciding between individuals. When we shift our attention away from choices between individuals and to the way in which we organize the health system, we can no longer rely on doctors and patients together arriving at some sort of tacit agreement about how needs are to be judged. Allocating health resources across a system requires a more explicit approach to the identification of need.

Different scholars have different approaches to the identification of need at a system level. Len Doyal (1995), for example, starts from the assumption that we can legitimately describe healthcare as a need, because good health is central to human flourishing. Not only do we need good health to do what we want to do with our lives for ourselves, we also need good health to be good citizens and help others fulfil their goals for themselves. Doyal argues that there are seven principles for the fair allocation of healthcare resources according to need. First, we should ration care within, rather than across different categories of treatment. To do this, first we need to work out the cost of the total demand for healthcare for a particular period of time. If the available funding is, say, 70% of this total, the fairest way to allocate is to cut healthcare services by 30% across the board. This criterion has been criticized because, in practice, it is difficult to allocate services neatly into one category or another. Is a weight-loss clinic, for example, an obesity service or a cardiovascular disease service? Doyal's criterion is also unavoidably backward looking as it is based on existing treatments and services. What if a new service becomes available? How do we incorporate it into our system?

Nonetheless, having made a certain amount of resources available within each category of care, we still have to decide between possible recipients. Doyal argues that we should rank individuals according to the impact that their illness or disability has on their capacity to flourish as human beings. Highest priority then goes to life-threatening illness, with lowest priority to treatments that we might like, but which do not really change our capacity to flourish (for example, some forms of cosmetic surgery). Many general practices do, in fact, have a system for allocating access to consultations that is something like this. A practice may have a one-hour block each morning to which patients who perceive an urgent need for medical treatment may come. For other, less urgent, conditions, there may be a waiting period of a few days before an appointment can be secured.

Box 7.3 Criteria for the allocation of healthcare resources according to need (from Doyal 1995)

1. Ration care within, rather than across, different categories of treatment.
2. Rank individuals according to the impact their illness or disability has on their capacity for human flourishing.
3. Randomize as a last resort.

Preconditions:

4. Do not spend scarce resources on ineffective treatments.
5. Lifestyle should not be relevant to our chances of getting the treatment we need.
6. Debate allocation issues openly and rationally.
7. There should be mechanisms to take account of the views of the community.

Once we have ranked people according to need, we may still be left having to choose between individuals. At this point, Doyal would advocate random allocation. Waiting lists are a form of random allocation, since there is some unpredictability about the moment that health problems strike us and prompt us to seek treatment.

Doyal's last four principles are really 'preconditions' (Butler 1999): we should not spend scarce resources on unproven treatments; lifestyle should not influence our chances of getting the treatment we need; we should debate allocation issues openly and rationally; and there should be mechanisms to take account of the views of the community.

Choosing between people on the basis of capacity to benefit

A second way to choose between people when allocating health resources is to focus on patients' capacity to benefit from a treatment. One of the reasons we decide not to pay for some interventions in some people is because it is considered unlikely that the person will receive any benefit from it. Sometimes this is an easy conclusion to reach; for example, a person with disseminated cancer and severe cardiovascular disease is very unlikely to benefit from a coronary artery bypass graft. However, most decisions are not clear-cut–patterns of health and illness are notoriously difficult to predict at an individual level and it can be impossible to say that a person will not get *any* benefit from a particular intervention. The increasing use of evidence-based medicine has led to more information about the statistical effectiveness of interventions, and this is increasingly used to control access to some services, but the question about the effectiveness in individuals remains. The phrase 'not clinically indicated' can mean a number of things: the intervention is not likely to benefit the patient or the use of the intervention in this patient is not considered a worthwhile use of resources (Mason and Laurie 2006). This kind of ambivalence can provide an indirect or perhaps easier way of refusing services, but may conceal the real reasons behind the refusal.

Evidence about the effectiveness of particular interventions has become increasingly influential through the activities of a number of organizations around the world that are charged with the preparation of reports on the effectiveness, efficiency and safety of new treatments in healthcare. Organizations such as the Canadian Agency for Drugs and Technologies in Health (CADTH) (Hailey 2007), the National Institute of Health and Clinical Excellence (NICE) in the United Kingdom (Walker *et al.* 2007), and the Pharmaceutical Benefits Advisory Committee (PBAC) and Medical Services Advisory Committee (MSAC) in Australia (Jackson 2007) play an important role in shaping access to health services. Their reports are used by healthcare providers as a basis for the preparation of clinical guidelines and the implementation of programmes and services. These reports also shape funding decisions in less direct ways, because they can provide the evidence that lobby groups may need to strengthen their case for (or against) the funding of certain services and stimulate debate about existing policies and guidelines (Hivon *et al.* 2005). It is not surprising, then, that there is often debate about the political nature of decisions made by these agencies, but the attempt to provide transparency in decisions about resource allocation is to be welcomed.

Studies of the effectiveness of various treatments in healthcare always include some assessment of patient capacity to benefit. The Quality Adjusted Life Year (QALY) is a measure that attempts to combine both the quantity and quality of life gained from a treatment in a single measure. The basic idea of a QALY is straightforward: one year of perfect health life expectancy is valued at 1; one year of less than perfect health life expectancy is valued at less than 1; and death is zero. A treatment that gives 6 months extra life at perfect health would be scored at 0.5, whereas a treatment giving 1 year of extra life in health that is only 25% of optimal health would be scored at 0.25. QALYs can provide an indication of the benefits gained from a variety of different medical procedures in terms of both quality of life and survival for the patient. The costs of different treatments can then be compared by looking at the costs per QALYs.

In theory, the use of QALYs can help in comparisons between competing treatments. For example, if a health service has £2 million to spend on new interventions, what kind of QALY gains can be expected from putting the money into hip replacements versus spending on asthma or coronary artery grafting? There has been much discussion about the uses and abuses of QALYs, and here we comment on two aspects. The first is apparent difficulties with economic information. If we look at just one example, that of estimating the cost-effectiveness of beta interferons and glatiramer acetate in the treatment of multiple sclerosis, the information is very confusing. Initial estimates of costs per QALY between 38,000 and 106,000 pounds almost double with methodological changes in the analysis, such as changes in the discount rates for costs and benefits (ScHARR 2001). These large variations indicate the lack of precision in economic estimates and the importance of methodological assumptions. Given the difficulties in ascribing accurate costs per QALY, it is concerning when decisions about resource allocation rely very heavily upon what may be fairly imprecise estimates.

Perhaps the more concerning problem with QALYs is the attempt to quantify the value of life in terms of degree of health. The assumption is that life in poor health is less worth living than life in perfect health. This assumption immediately discriminates against people with any kind of disability or chronic health problem, as they cannot gain the same QALY benefit from an intervention as a person without disability or chronic illness. Each person's life is valuable to him or herself, even if they are not in perfect health. The question posed by QALYs seems unanswerable except at a personal level, and even at this level it is hard to imagine how a choice could be made: how would you value 1 year of life at 50% health (whatever that means) compared with 6 months at full health?

Choosing between people on the basis of merit or desert

A third way to choose between people when health services are scarce is to focus on merit or desert as a criterion. When we speak of people deserving or meriting things, we imply that their contribution, effort or status is important and ought to be taken into account when resources are allocated. On the face of it, this seems a reprehensible way to allocate health services. Surely we ought not to give people preferential treatment just because they are wealthy or a member of parliament or a promising young gymnast! However, as we shall see, the merit criterion often plays a role when health services are rationed and, sometimes, it is hard to argue against its place.

Box 7.4 Examples of merit-based criteria for the allocation of healthcare resources

Criteria related to character:

+ grateful patients;
+ compliant patients.

Criteria related to social role:

+ past role (e.g. World War II Veteran);
+ present role (e.g. single mother with dependent children);
+ future role (e.g. a young person).

There are a number of ways we can conceive of merit or desert operating as a criterion for allocating healthcare. First, we can imagine allocating healthcare to people according to their personal appeal or characteristics. Should personality traits be relevant to the allocation of healthcare resources? There is always the temptation in general practice to focus attention on patients who are appropriately grateful for what we do for them. Personal appeal ought to be morally unacceptable, but it sometimes turns out to be the reason we treat people differently. Ethical stewarding of resources in general practice attempts to guard against such behaviour.

It is easy to show that allocating resources in general practice on the basis of how 'nice' people are is not acceptable and should not occur. However, it gets a bit harder when the character traits become 'being cooperative' or 'trying hard'. Patients' interest in, and capacity to comply with, treatment does have a practical influence on how much call they have on scarce healthcare services. For example, should a GP encourage a 42-year-old overweight smoker with asthma to join the practice Stop Smoking Clinic, even when he knows that all advice just goes in one ear and out the other? According to a needs-based argument, this patient needs the GP's time and support far more than other, more compliant, patients do. A character-based allocation of resources may be behind Dr Schroeder's consultation with Jennifer. Jennifer may just happen to be a reserved, quiet person who does not offer much information but, if invited, is willing to talk. Should reticent patients be discriminated against because they find it harder to raise problems with their GP? To what extent does Dr Schroeder have an obligation to make it as easy for Jennifer to discuss her problems as it is for a more garrulous, extroverted patient?

The problem with this version of merit-based resource allocation is that it is rather difficult to put together an argument for treating people differently, based purely on their character. As Butler suggests, the case for treating nice (or responsive or extroverted) people preferentially rests upon the assumption that they have, in some sense, done something that ought to be rewarded or, at least, not punished (Butler 1999, p.52). The idea of allocating resources according to desert makes sense only when people can do something to influence their desert, rather like training hard to win the prize at the end of a race. But, people are often unable to influence those characteristics that seem to make them deserving or undeserving of healthcare. The real problem with this version of the merit criterion is that the link between character, actions and free will is actually very complex. Continuing smoking, for example, is more than a personal choice. It is also a result of clever advertising, peer pressure and the extremely addictive qualities of nicotine. In addition, smoking-related illness often strikes in life at a point far removed from the decision to take up smoking. How much responsibility should people have to bear for decisions they may have made decades earlier?

There is a second way in which merit-based criteria for the allocation of health resources can be interpreted. This involves considering the social roles that people play and taking these roles into account when resources are allocated. Here, we can take into account people's current role, their past contribution or their potential for contribution in the future.

We can think of examples that would fit each category. For example, if we are thinking about people's current role, we might argue that, all other things being equal, a mother with three dependent children should take priority over 35-year-old bachelor, when it comes to access to health services. If we take into account people's past contribution, this would allow us to discriminate in favour of people who have in the past contributed significantly to society, perhaps through their service to the community, or their work as a distinguished scientist. Finally, if we look ahead to the future, we may discriminate against the elderly in favour of the young, on the basis that the young are likely to benefit society in years to come whereas the elderly have little to offer.

Such judgements are sometimes pounced on by the media. For example, there have been a number of celebrated cases in the United Kingdom where decisions about access to scarce, often expensive, treatment appear to have been made on the basis of social roles. While this may seem to be a long way from general practice, there are many situations in which social role does influence resource allocation in general practice settings. For example, some surgeries limit the time that parents with young children wait before they see the GP, implying that there is something about being a child that is relevant to your access to the GP. Or, patients who can afford it may be encouraged to pay extra for quick access to services about which poorer patients are not necessarily informed.

Introducing these alternatives reframes the question of the merit criterion as one of the place of social contribution in decision-making about resource allocation. Again, in this arena, the tricky issues of free will and responsibility rear their heads. Just how able are we to make ourselves socially valuable people? Issues such as these are inevitably controversial, and explicit discussion of them is often swept under the carpet. The point we wish to make here is that merit criteria for resource allocation are often used unconsciously or appear disguised as other reasons. Such a situation is undesirable. If we are to use such social worth criteria, the debate about their applicability needs to occur in the open and in a constructive manner.

Choosing between people on the basis of rights

There is a lot of talk about a 'right to healthcare'–much of it rather confusing. What does it mean to say that people have a right to healthcare? Does having a right to healthcare include having a right to cosmetic surgery because you think, as Simone does, that your nose is unattractive? Or is having a right to healthcare having only a right to emergency surgery? What about Mr Servante's right to have his questions answered fully?

In many of the countries in which general practice plays a key gatekeeping role, such as the United Kingdom, Australia, the Netherlands or Canada, debate about the right to healthcare has usually played second fiddle to discussion of clinical need. This is because health systems such as the National Health Service in the UK have been based on the core principle that they 'will provide a universal service for all based on clinical need, not ability to pay' (National Health Service 2000). This is not necessarily the case in other countries, notably in the United States of America, in which debate about resource allocation tends to focus mainly on rights. Still, it is important to introduce the concept of a right to healthcare here, if only in brief.

We are born with some rights. For example, there are rights to be allowed to do things, to be free of interference (for example, rights to life, liberty and property). There are also rights to be given things (for example, rights to employment and subsistence, food, clothing, housing or medical care). Such rights are the content of statements such as the Universal Declaration of Human Rights.

There is a second kind of right that is linked more closely to the way the society we live in is organized. Some rights are acquired through agreements, contracts or promises that we are party to. These contracts or promises can take a variety of forms, from those which have the full force of the law behind them (for example, my right as a pedestrian to expect cars to stop for me at pedestrian crossings is protected by traffic laws) to those that are merely established forms of behaviour, where no explicit promises have been made (for example, the right of a child to care and concern by her parents). When patients attend a general practice, they have a right to receive primary care from that practice, and behind this right sits the agreements that the staff of the practice have made with the funder of the service, whether that be the patient, a health insurer or government.

There is usually, to some degree, a right to healthcare in both of the senses identified above. We can describe the right to healthcare as a basic right. The difficulty with thinking about a right in this way is that it does not make clear just who is obligated to attend to the right to healthcare. The person or persons with the obligation to provide care remain shadowy characters, sometimes taking the form of 'the government' or 'the health authority'.

To be clear about who is obliged to provide the service, we need to turn to our second definition of a right. If we focus on a right to healthcare as a contract or promise, then it is easier to identify the individuals and groups who have a duty to provide healthcare. For GPs, this issue is most relevant in the context of their relationship with the patients who attend their practice. Many practices have a statement of patient rights, which will include such things as:

- Confidentiality from all members of staff.
- Courteous treatment by all staff.
- Access to personal medical records.
- An appointment the same day for acute illnesses.
- An appointment within a week for non-acute illnesses.
- Complaints mechanisms that are enforced.

With respect to these rights, the obligation to meet patient expectations lies with the GPs and other practice staff. Implicit in these statements is the assumption that all patients registered with the practice have the same right of access to services.

Conclusion

In this chapter we have explored a range of issues that arise because of the problem of scarcity in healthcare. We have reviewed the range of ways in which resource allocation decisions are made in the NHS and considered the four main contenders for a just allocation of health resources—allocation according to need, to capacity to benefit, to merit and to rights. Our discussion of these issues grew out of the consideration of the principle of beneficence in Chapter 6. In the next chapter we return to issues more directly concerned with the care of individual patients, with a discussion of patient autonomy in general practice.

References

Butler J (1999). *The ethics of healthcare rationing. Principles and practices*. Cassell, London.

Daniels N and Sabin J (1997). Limits to healthcare: fair procedures, democratic deliberation, and the legitimacy problem for insurers. *Philosophy and Public Affairs* **26**, 303–350.

Daniels N (2000). Accountability for reasonableness. Establishing a fair process for priority setting is easier than agreeing on principles. *British Medical Journal* **321**(7272), 1300–1301.

Doyal L (1995). Needs, rights and equity, moral quality in healthcare rationing. *Quality in Healthcare* **4**, 273–283.

Hailey DM (2007). Health technology assessment in Canada, diversity and evolution. *Medical Journal of Australia* **187**, 286–288.

Hivon M, Lehoux P, Denis J-L and Tailliez S (2005). Use of health technology assessment in decision making, Coresponsibility of users and producers? *International Journal of Technology Assessment in Healthcare* **21**, 268–275.

Jackson TJ (2007). Health technology assessment in Australia: challenges ahead. *Medical Journal of Australia* **187**, 262–264.

Mason JK and Laurie GT (2006). *Mason and McCall Smith's law and medical ethics* (7th edn). Oxford University Press, Oxford.

Medical Services Advisory Committee (2008). Medical Services Advisory Committee, Strengthening evidence-based healthcare in Australia. Australian Government Department of Health and Ageing. Available at http: //www.msac.gov.au/ (accessed 14 January 2008).

National Health Service (2000). *Your guide to the NHS*. Available at http: //www.nhs.uk/ (accessed 25 August 2008).

Newdick C (2004). *Who should we treat? Rights, rationing and resources in the NHS* (2nd edn). Oxford University Press, Oxford, 93–128.

Rawls J (1972). *A theory of justice*. Oxford University Press, Oxford..

ScHARR (2001). *Cost effectiveness of beta interferons and glatiramer acetate in the management of multiple sclerosis*. Final report to the National Institute for Clinical Excellence. Sheffield, ScHARR. Avalable at http: //www.nice.org.uk/pdf/msscharrreport.pdf

van de Ven WPMM (1995). Choices in healthcare, a contribution from the Netherlands. *British Medical Bulletin* **51**, 781–790.

van der Grinten TED and Kasdorp JP (1999). Choices in Dutch healthcare, mixing strategies and responsibilities *Health Policy* **50**, 105–122.

Walker S, Palmer S and Sculpher M (2007). The role of NICE technology appraisal in NHS rationing. *British Medical Bulletin* **81** and **82**, 51–64. DOI, 10.1093/bmb/ldm007.

Chapter 8

Making decisions: patient autonomy in general practice

Introduction

Case 8.1

Grace Hopkins is a 54-year-old woman with mild to moderate osteoarthritis of both knees, for which she takes regular non-steroidal anti-inflammatories. Grace also has a past history of a meniscal tear followed by arthroscopy for partial removal of cartilage in her right knee. She comes to see her GP, Dr Amy Walker, for medical advice prior to going trekking for 3 weeks in Nepal. Grace wishes to know what the likely effect of the trekking will be, and if there is anything that she can do to minimize the damage to her knees. Dr Walker thinks that the trekking will accelerate the arthritis and that Grace will return with swollen and painful knees, which may take months to settle down to their present state. The trip may increase the likelihood of Grace needing early knee replacements. From a medical point of view, trekking will be harmful to Grace's musculo-skeletal health. Dr Walker explains this to Grace, who then goes away to think it over. Later she tells Dr Walker that she will be going trekking, as this has been one of her goals for many years and she thinks this is her last opportunity. She understands that her knees will suffer, but thinks the overall value and meaning of the trip are worth any subsequent ill effects.

In this scenario, Grace has sought medical advice to help her make a decision with health implications. She accepted the prediction that her knees will be harmed, but decided to go ahead with the trip. We might not have made the same decision in her place, but we can understand her right to make this decision, and we can recognize that this is very much her decision, based upon a thoughtful consideration of the risks and benefits to her. In ethical terms, we describe decisions like this as autonomous, reflecting the wishes and values of the person involved and in some important way, belonging to that person rather than being imposed by external forces.

What is autonomy and why is it important?

Autonomy can be a tricky term to define or understand. We can describe people, decisions or actions as autonomous. An autonomous person shapes and directs his or her own life, based upon their own values, to bring about their own choices and plans (Young 2001). Autonomous actions or decisions reflect a person's full understanding and evaluation of the relevant issues, taking place in a voluntary way without any coercion or manipulation. The idea of free action, not being coerced or forced by anyone else, is central to understanding autonomy. Much of our thinking about autonomy has been influenced by JS Mill (Box 8.1).

Box 8.1 The liberty principle

Over himself, over his own body and mind, the individual is sovereign.

Exception to the principle:
The only purpose for which power can be rightfully exercised over any member of a civilised community, against his will, is to prevent harm to others. His own good, either physical or moral, is not a sufficient warrant.

(Mill 1991, p.14)

Why did Mill think that personal autonomy is so important? Is it because autonomy is valuable for itself, or because things are likely to turn out better if people are left alone to make their own decisions? The second reason is straightforward to understand: things are likely to turn out better if people make their own decisions because:

- individuals are the best placed to know and understand what is important to them–they are the best judge of their own interests;
- individuals are more likely than anyone else to be motivated to try to get what is best for themselves;
- people resent interference, even well meaning interference, so it may be counterproductive to force people into a course of action even if it is for their own good.

As well as these consequentialist reasons, autonomy is important for itself because being autonomous expresses aspects of being human that we value highly, like the capacity to make decisions that reflect our uniqueness as individuals and the capacity to develop in ways that foster our particular character traits and interests. Without the freedom to be autonomous, we would lose much of our individuality (Christie and Hoffmaster 1986; Kultgen 1995).

Autonomy in practice

In ethical terms, we recognize the importance of personal autonomy through the obligation that doctors have to respect the autonomy of patients. The principle of respect for patients' autonomy protects the right that patients have to control their own bodies and to make their own decisions about medical treatment. Respecting patient autonomy means that doctors should not examine patients or give treatments unless the patient has given their informed consent for this to happen.

Historically speaking, the idea that patients should be autonomous with regard to their medical care is a relatively recent phenomenon, emerging from the 1960s in the wake of civil rights movements. As discussed in Chapter 6, the idea that doctors are experts because of their medical knowledge runs deep, and this expertise is often used as a justification for doctors to make decisions for patients. As well as historical precedent, there are practical reasons for thinking that patients either may not want to, or be able to, make their own decisions about medical care, for various reasons. Despite these reservations, the principle of respect for patient autonomy has become one of the central planks of contemporary medical ethics, with the practice of informed consent serving as a legal reminder of its importance. Later in the chapter we will look at some of the practicalities and implications for the doctor–patient relationship of the duty to respect patient autonomy.

Before discussing informed consent in detail, it is worth considering what we mean by 'respect'. How can doctors show that they respect the right of their patients to make their own decisions, even if they disagree with the decision? Respecting another person involves recognizing that that person has a unique nature with their own feelings and desires, and the capacity to work out what is best for themselves (Downie and Calman 1994). Respect also involves practical aspects, such as maintaining confidentiality (see Chapter 5) and protecting patient privacy, as well as using a courteous manner and addressing people in their preferred way. The process of respecting is important; in the scenario at the beginning of the chapter we did not spell out how Dr Walker actually replied to Grace's enquiry. She may have explained her prognosis in a sympathetic way that expressed her understanding of the importance of the trip and the need for Grace to have as much information as possible to make her decision. Or Dr Walker may have responded in a bullying or derisive way, implying that trekking was a ridiculous idea and that Grace would need extra medical care as a result. Respect requires us to understand the impact both of what we are saying and the way we are saying it, avoiding patronizing expression and judgmental assumptions.

Informed consent

Informed consent is a mechanism for people to control what happens to them, forming an important part of respecting autonomy. The main aim of informed consent is to ensure that people are acting freely, without coercion or deception (O'Neill 2003). Informed consent is the process through which people can authorize what happens to them or who touches them; this process makes medical treatments morally acceptable in most circumstances. The law strongly supports this moral position: before you can examine, treat or care for a competent adult person, you must obtain their informed consent in most jurisdictions. Without consent, touching a patient or taking blood is potential battery, even if the action is intended to help rather than harm the patient (Mason and Laurie 2006).

In general practice, consent is often taken for granted. There are no forms to sign as for surgery, and patients are usually considered to consent to their care by the fact of turning up. But this does not decrease the moral importance of making sure that patients make informed decisions about their own care. How can we tell when or if consent is informed? The conditions for informed consent try to ensure that any decision the patient makes is autonomous by asking three questions:

- Is this person competent to make the decision?
- Do they understand the necessary information?
- Are they making the decision freely?

Competence

Competence is to do with the ability of a person to make decisions that reflect their values and their concern for their own wellbeing, or in other words, their *capacity* to make autonomous decisions (Young 2001). How can we tell if a person is competent to make a decision, especially if it is one that we have difficulty understanding?

Case 8.2

Paul McKinney is a 34-year-old patient with schizophrenia. He takes long-acting psychotropic medication for his schizophrenia, which has been

Case 8.2 *(continued)*

well-controlled for the past few months, with the exception of some fixed paranoid delusions about the media. Dr Jeremy Chu is called to do a house visit because Paul has had 24 hours of severe abdominal pain. On examination, Paul is febrile and has the clinical signs of appendicitis. Dr Chu explains the diagnosis in terms of part of the bowel being infected, with the risk of rupturing, and the possible consequences if this occurs. He recommends to Paul that he go straight to the local emergency department for observation and possible operation. Paul seems to understand what Dr Chu is saying and the risks of not going to hospital, but he says that he will not go to the hospital because he dislikes the way that they treat him there, he does not want an operation and he wants to see if he can recover with treatment from Dr Chu.

Is this a competent decision? Dr Chu is in a difficult position, as he thinks it is very much in Paul's best interests to go to the hospital, but at the same time, Paul seems to understand the risks. Paul fulfils the criteria for competence, as he can understand what is proposed, the benefits and risks, and make a decision based upon his values and preferences (see Box 8.2).

Box 8.2 Assessing capacity to consent to or refuse treatment

1. Is the person able to understand information about the medical condition and any proposed treatment including:
   - what the treatment is and why it is being proposed;
   - the main benefits and risks;
   - any alternatives that are available;
   - the consequences of not accepting the treatment.
2. Is the patient able to comprehend and retain relevant information, so that they can reason and deliberate about the options, taking into account other considerations?
3. Are they able to make a choice consistent with their value and goals?
4. Is their choice maintained over time?
5. Can they communicate their choice to the doctor?

(Adapted from McMillan and Tan 2004; Derse 2005)

Unlike the decision made by Grace in the first example, it is much harder to understand Paul's decision. A dislike of hospitals hardly seems a good enough reason to refuse potentially life-saving treatment. Yet, as long as Paul's decision is competent, it does not matter how irrational or wrong it seems to others, there is no moral or legal basis for compelling him to go to hospital. Difficult though it may be, Dr Chu has to accept Paul's decision, as well as ongoing responsibility for Paul's medical care, guided by the interventions that he will accept.

Despite Paul's schizophrenia, he is competent to make this decision about treatment for appendicitis, as he can understand the nature of appendicitis and the likely consequences of his decision, and has weighed up this information against his reasons for not wishing to go to hospital. In practice, competence is assessed relative to the decision at hand. Doctors usually have a higher threshold for determining competence as the consequences become more severe. This makes sense, as we consider consequences to be ethically significant and, if the potential harms are serious, we have a stronger duty to make sure that the person is capable of making the decision. Ethics and law, however, may part company here as legal capacity is either present or absent, irrespective of the gravity of the decision (Buchanan 2004).

Case 8.2 continued

With Paul's consent, Dr Chu discusses Paul's condition with the surgical registrar and treats him with a dose of antibiotics. When he visits the next morning, Paul is worse, with obvious dehydration and signs of peritonitis. Dr Chu once again explains what has happened and stresses that without fluid replacement and further antibiotics, Paul is at risk of dying.

This time Paul agrees to admission.

We tend to think of consent as a one-off event, either the patient refuses or consents to treatment. However, patients have a right to review their decision and alter it, in the light of changing circumstances. We may not know why Paul changed his mind, but Dr Chu had an obligation to keep checking Paul's decision, and to keep the channels of communication open in case he revised his decision. The ongoing nature of consent is important as people's views about a treatment may well change after they have experienced for themselves the side-effects or benefits over time.

Understanding

One of the conditions for autonomous decisions is that the person concerned understands the full implications of their decision. This is perhaps the hardest condition to come to grips with–how much information does a patient need to understand fully the possible consequences of their decision, and how can a doctor make sure that the patient is both informed and understands this information?

To understand, in a medical situation, the patient needs to actually comprehend the language used by the doctor and then be able to relate that information to their own circumstances. How do we judge whether or not understanding has been achieved? From the patient's perspective, the language of medicine is often foreign and difficult to interpret in terms of knowing what is significant and what is not. In the process of becoming a doctor, a person doubles his or her vocabulary (Rogers 1992). This means that a large proportion of the words doctors use are unfamiliar to the general population.

A certain amount of knowledge is necessary before a patient can understand the relevance of what is being said. A patient may feel that they have enough information to make a decision, but it is probably only in retrospect that they can properly judge whether or not they did understand what their treatment would really be like. Research suggests that when people are asked in retrospect about the information they were given about a treatment, 40 to 60% of patients do not understand the purpose of their treatment, and 45% cannot recall any major risks or complications (Cassileth *et al.* 1980; Olver *et al.* 1994; Cox 2001).

One problem with understanding is the difference between understanding what will happen and actually knowing what that will feel like. A side-effect of nocturnal diuresis, affecting 30–40% of people who take a particular drug, may sound acceptable to a patient, but after 3 weeks of interrupted sleep, the patient may realize that this is unacceptable to them.

Another problem with understanding is the inherently uncertain nature of medicine. Despite their best efforts, doctors are not able to accurately predict what will happen in each case. If a person suffers a rare side-effect from treatment, although they may have been aware that this was possible, it is not clear that this is the same as understanding that it might actually happen to them, and what it would be like if it did happen.

Case 8.3

Glenn Wattie is a 56-year-old man, who visits Dr Mackenzie fairly infrequently. One day he comes in to see Dr Mackenzie requesting a test for

Case 8.3 *(continued)*

prostate cancer. His uncle has just been diagnosed with disseminated prostate cancer, and Glenn Wattie wants a test to make sure that the same thing does not happen to him.

How much information does Glenn need to make an informed decision about the prostate cancer test, and how well can he understand the potential risks of the situation while he is distressed about his uncle and clinging to the belief that the test is necessary to 'prevent him from getting cancer'? Dr Mackenzie needs time to explain the nature of screening tests, and the difference between screening and prevention. Glenn cannot give his informed consent for the test until he understands the benefits and potential harms. Sometimes it seems easier and quicker to do the test rather than explain all the pros and cons to the patient, but adopting this course of action ignores the moral obligation to respect the autonomy of patients. We know that patients have a strong desire for information (Ende *et al.* 1989; Ong *et al.* 1995; Charles *et al.* 1997) and that doctors consistently under-estimate this (Sullivan *et al.* 2001).

There are no set rules for judging how much information a doctor should give to a patient. From the moral point of view, the aim is to ensure that the patient has all of the information that they need to make an autonomous decision, which means tailoring the information to the interests and concerns of that patient. This is a demanding requirement, and one that is time-consuming to fulfil. However, in general practice, it may be easier to reach this standard than in branches of secondary or tertiary care for a couple of reasons. General practice allows an ongoing relationship in which information may be exchanged over time, and the GP may know the patient well enough to be able to 'fit' the information to the patient in a meaningful way. Patients in general practice can come to know their GP's communication style, and to trust that the GP knows them well enough to explain the important and relevant information and omit the rest.

From a legal point of view, a doctor who does not give their patient enough information may be considered negligent. There are different standards for judging how much information is enough in different jurisdictions. For example, UK law generally uses a professional standard to judge negligence, although recent common law developments are modifying this (see Mason and Laurie 2006; Chapter 9). This means that the information that you tell the patient has to be within the boundaries of acceptable practice (i.e. what at least some doctors usually tell patients) as judged by a responsible body of medical opinion. This is known as the Bolam ruling or standard.

However, the courts do recognize the importance of doctors disclosing *all* risks that may be relevant to that specific patient, irrespective of usual professional practice. This means using the patient's perspective rather than that of the medical profession. This standard is known as the material risk or prudent patient standard; it is ethically preferable to the professional standard, as this is more likely to help the patient to make a fully informed decision. The material risk standard operates in other jurisdictions, such as Australia, following the famous Rogers and Whitaker case. Here the court defined a risk as material if:

> … in the circumstances of the particular case, a reasonable [or ordinary] person in the patient's position, if warned of the risk, would be likely to attach significance to it or if the medical practitioner is or should be reasonably aware that the particular patient, if warned of the risk, would be likely to attach significance to it.

> (Cited at Skene 2004, p.175)

The responsibility lies with the doctor to decide what information is material to the particular patient, taking into account (Skene 2004, p.180):

- the nature of the matter to be disclosed;
- the nature of the treatment;
- the desire of the patient for information;
- the temperament and health of the patient;
- the general circumstances.

Is it ever justified for doctors to withhold information from patients? One reason that is suggested for withholding information is the fear of self-fulfilling prophecies in relation to the prognosis or treatment (Christie and Hoffmaster 1986). If a patient who has just been prescribed beta-blockers, for example, is told that one of the side-effects is tiredness, this may create the expectation in that patient that they will feel tired. This is a bit like the placebo effect but, instead of feeling better because that is what is expected, the patient experiences the side-effect because this is what they are expecting. Is there an ethical way to minimize the placebo effect for side-effects without deliberately withholding information? Different GPs have different ways of explaining side-effects, and patients have varying desires for information, making it hard to generalize. One option is to review the patient at an early time and ask if they have experienced any side-effects, leaving it up to the patient to identify any unusual or new experiences, which the GP may then confirm. However, this can leave the patient not knowing what to expect and potentially distressed by seemingly unexplained symptoms. Decisions as to how much information about side-effects to tell patients require judgement, based upon the GP's knowledge of the patient and the frequency and severity of the possible side-effects. If a patient asks about the nature of any side-effects, the doctor is obliged to respond honestly.

A second reason for withholding information is if a doctor believes that the information will seriously harm a patient's health or welfare. This is known as therapeutic privilege. The conditions in which doctors may exercise therapeutic privilege are extremely limited, given the strong moral imperative to provide patients with information and the dangers of paternalism. There must be a risk of serious harm to the patient, and not just the inconvenience of the patient disagreeing with the doctor or making an apparently unwise choice. There must also be reasonable grounds for the doctor to believe that the patient will be harmed significantly by the information; for example, from past experience with this patient or others in similar situations.

There are also pragmatic reasons why GPs might withhold information, the most obvious being lack of time. This is a constant pressure, trying to meet the needs of individual patients for information while also meeting overall patient demand (see also Chapter 7). In Chapter 3 we discussed the importance of trust in the doctor–patient relationship, and it is worth referring back to this in the context of giving information to patients, to pose the question: What does this patient trust me to do, and how much am I expecting them to trust my judgement in this case? In a doctor–patient relationship character-ized by trust, it is possible to develop mutual short-cuts; for example, the patient might ask, 'Is there is anything that you think I should know about this treatment?' trusting the GP to tailor information to their specific circumstances. Conversely, GPs need a certain amount of trust in their patients to provide enough information for patients to make informed choices. Trust smoothes the process for patients to have some control over decision-making.

Another reason why GPs might withhold information is because of discom-fort over the issues that might be raised. This typically occurs in relation to disclosing bad news about poor prognoses, when the GP might be faced with discussing the impending death of the patient. (See Chapter 11 for specific discussion of end-of-life issues.) Recent research from the US indicates a sig-nificant gap between patients' desire for information about serious diagnoses and physicians' estimates of these. Only 42% of physicians said patients want to be told all details about a serious illness; 57% said patients want to be told only in general terms; and 1% said patients want no information. However, up to 82% of patients wanted to be told all the details, with this percentage drop-ping to 61% for patients over 60 years of age (Sullivan *et al.* 2001). GPs may feel uncomfortable breaking bad news and discussing death, but this is not a morally acceptable reason for withholding information.

Discussions about informed consent can become side-tracked into concerns over the extent of information to be disclosed, or how much persuasion is acceptable, and whether or not the patient is making the decision. At times it is worth standing back to remember the ethical point at stake, which is that it is wrong to deceive or coerce people, as this prevents them from making autonomous choices. Information is a means to this: if a patient receives explanations so that she is able to understand the implications of accepting or refusing a treatment, she is then in a position to make a choice if she wishes to. The obligation of doctors is to promote or protect the capacity of the patient for autonomous action by providing enough information so that the patient has the opportunity to make a meaningful decision.

Voluntariness

The final condition for autonomous decisions is voluntariness: to be autonomous, a person's decision should not be manipulated or coerced in any way, by a health professional, by relatives or anyone else.

Case 8.4

Mrs Butler is an elderly woman who lives alone, with weekly visits from her daughter. One day her daughter, Alice, makes an appointment for Mrs Butler to see her GP, Dr Singh. In the consultation, Alice says that her mother has not been well lately. She has no appetite and has lost weight. Alice would like Dr Singh to examine Mrs Butler and do some tests, to find out what is wrong. Mrs Butler is silent for most of the consultation, and when asked if she is willing to have an examination, her daughter answers 'Of course'.

During the examination, Dr Singh asks Alice to leave the room. Mrs Butler has a large craggy mass in her left breast and an enlarged liver. Dr Singh tells Mrs Butler that there is something wrong in her breast and says that she would need to do some tests to find out exactly what it is, but that it may be cancer. She asks if she is willing to have the tests. At this stage Alice comes back into the room, wanting to know what the examination has shown and what tests Dr Singh is going to do. Dr Singh again asks Alice to leave the room, but she insists that her mother wants her there, appealing to Mrs Butler for confirmation. Mrs Butler nods her head and asks the doctor to explain things to Alice. Dr Singh outlines the situation and Alice says, 'Of course Mum wants the tests, when can they be done?'.

Dr Singh is worried that Alice is coercing Mrs Butler into this consultation and the investigations, and that she does not know what Mrs Butler would really like to happen.

Discussions about autonomy can give the impression that it is easy to distinguish between a decision that is voluntary and one that is coerced in some way but, in reality, the distinction can be tricky. From the information in this scenario, Mrs Butler appears to be pressured, if not bullied, by her daughter. For Dr Singh, the task is to find out Mrs Butler's own preferences, starting with her knowledge of Mrs Butler based upon their existing relationship. Maybe Mrs Butler always looks to her daughter for guidance and most of her medical care occurs through the agency of the daughter. On the other hand, maybe Mrs Butler has mentioned in previous consultations that if she gets a potentially terminal illness, she would not want to have any treatment, or that she finds her daughter over-interfering. Dr Singh cannot be sure of Mrs Butler's own preferences about investigation and treatment until she has had a chance to talk to her on her own. Arranging this may involve some subterfuge on her part, but it is essential to find out this information.

This case raises a wider point about the decisions that people make. We have said that to be autonomous a decision must in some way belong to that person, to be in character rather than be directed by another. However, humans are social creatures, living in relationships with others whose views we respect and whose advice we seek, especially when we need to make serious decisions. People *are* influenced by the wishes and desires of others, and responding to those influences strengthens and deepens our relationships. Does this somehow limit or damage personal autonomy? If we consider that having meaningful relationships is an important part of what people wish for themselves, then we have to look at autonomy in a broader sense than that of purely individualistic decision-making. If people are free to choose or maintain their relationships, then accepting advice and being influenced within those freely chosen relationships may not compromise autonomy at all. Relationships contribute to who people are, so that part of being 'in character' is to make decisions with input from others, in the context of significant relationships.

How can we accept this view of autonomy without losing the requirement for voluntariness? We need to consider the context of decision-making, and the relationship between the person making the decision and those around them. Cases at either end of the spectrum will be easy to identify; for example, a woman brought to the GP by an overbearing partner for a referral for tubal ligation that she does not want is being coerced in an unacceptable way. On the other hand, an elderly parent brought for a check up by a concerned son, in a way that reflects the long-standing dynamics of their relationship, can be an example of acceptable influence and persuasion.

Doctors have a responsibility to use all available information to work out what is going on in each situation, by asking questions like:

- Why does this patient have her relative with her?
- Is this the decision that I would have expected in this situation?
- Whose interests are being met by this decision?
- Does the patient seem comfortable with this choice?

Any pre-existing doctor–patient relationship is an invaluable resource, especially if the GP knows what kinds of things the patient usually trusts him to do.

Is illness itself coercive? In some sense it is, as when we are ill we do all sorts of things that we would prefer not to, like having blood tests or taking medication. But although illness narrows our range of choices, illness itself is not considered coercive in the same way as controlling actions taken by other people. Illness happens by chance, making it morally neutral. We cannot rationally blame another individual for making us ill, in the same way that we could blame someone who coerced us by holding a gun to our head. Human actions and their consequences can be judged on a moral scale, but events like illness that occur irrespective of human action cannot be judged on the same scale. Having said this, there are circumstances in which other individuals are to blame for ill health—for example, bio-terrorism attacks or exposure to dangerous agents—and the known links between socio-economic status and health care create a moral imperative for societies to act to reduce preventable ill health.

Doctors and other health professionals can be sources of manipulation or undue persuasion, either consciously or unconsciously. In theory, voluntary informed consent involves the patient making a selection between alternative courses of action, having received information about these from a doctor. Ideally the doctor should present relevant information in a neutral manner, so that the patient can choose the best option for themselves, rather than being influenced by the preferences of the doctor. However, it can be difficult for doctors to present information in an entirely neutral manner. Often the doctor does think that one course of action is better than another, and it may be hard to conceal this view. The way the information is presented can have a significant effect on the patient's view about a treatment. Usually we describe the benefits of a proposed course of treatment before describing the side-effects or complications. Framing information in a positive way encourages an initial commitment to the treatment before the full extent of any disadvantages are apparent (Cialdini *et al.* 1978; Faden and Beauchamp 1986) and has been found to influence patients' choices in practice (Cox 2001). Once the psychological commitment has been made, people are less likely to withdraw their consent, even when faced with quite significant drawbacks. Is this a form of acceptable persuasion or unacceptable manipulation?

It is important to keep sight of any motives the doctor has for suggesting one particular course of action over another. Strong persuasion or unintentional manipulation motivated by beneficence is more acceptable than actions motivated by, for example, personal gain, such as persuading a patient to enter a drug trial so that the GP will receive payment (see Chapter 12 for a full discussion of conflicts of interest). Patients attend GPs for medical advice and treatment, providing some prima-facie justification for GPs to put the medical case quite strongly, within the bounds of avoiding deception and bullying. Patients who disagree with the medical model of illness and its associated values are free to seek healthcare from alternative and complementary practitioners (within the limits of their personal resources). However, doctors may be influenced by other factors that are not necessarily known to patients, such as religious beliefs. For example, a GP with a strong belief in the sanctity of life may believe it is wrong to refer a woman for a termination of pregnancy, and do his best to dissuade her. In situations where GPs' personal beliefs influence their clinical decisions, GPs have an obligation to make their beliefs explicit, or to refer the patient to another practitioner.

Limits on autonomy and difficult cases

Case 8.5

Elsie Butterworth is a 68-year-old woman with alcoholism. She drinks to dangerous levels, has had a number of serious falls and is likely to die from her disease. Dr Buchan has seen Elsie on numerous occasions and each time informs her of the dangers of her current levels of drinking and the need to undergo some kind of rehabilitation. Elsie acknowledges the dangers and seems to agree that she should do something about her drinking, but each time she fails to keep appointments and her drinking does not diminish. Dr Buchan thinks that Elsie is not acting autonomously, because of her alcohol addiction. It would be in her best interests to receive treatment, but Dr Buchan is not able to admit Elsie for compulsory treatment, as the relevant legislation specifically excludes compulsory treatment solely for substance abuse.

GPs are often faced with patients who do not seem autonomous due to addiction or psychological disorders, but who cannot receive compulsory treatment based upon their best interests, because they do not meet the criteria for compulsory treatment under the relevant mental health legislation. How can the GP fulfil his or her ethical obligations in these situations? In general, mental health legislation tries to strike a balance between protecting people who are incapacitated by mental illness and, at the same time, protecting the rights of people to refuse unwanted treatment. This is always going to be a difficult balance that leaves some patients who are not able to make autonomous decisions, perhaps due to psychological compulsions, outside the jurisdiction of the legislation. For GPs the task can seem both endless and thankless, fruitlessly repeating the same advice, with the same lack of effect, while the patient becomes worse. It is important to recognize the GP's lack of agency in these situations: GPs do not have the power to intervene in terms of compulsory treatment for the patient's good except in very limited circumstances (see below). Acknowledgement that changing the situation is beyond the control of the GP can help to ease frustration and open the way for looking at ethical responses. The GP has ongoing obligations to maintain a respectful relationship with the patient and to offer such care as the patient is able or willing to accept. Building up a relationship may eventually lead to change for the patient, but at the very least, an ongoing relationship offers the best chance of minimising further harm to the patient.

Sometimes it is possible to develop creative solutions with patients, protecting long-term patient autonomy through periods of diminished capacity.

Case 8.6

Ian Johnson is a 32-year-old lawyer with established bi-polar disease. When he becomes manic, he is very articulate and persuasive, and it has been very difficult to admit him for compulsory treatment. He has had prolonged periods of mania during which he refused treatment. This has led to serious consequences for his personal life, employment and financial security. After one episode of mania, he asked his GP, Dr McFarlane, to help him to avoid similar situations in the future. Ian arranged an advance directive that authorizes Dr McFarlane to arrange compulsory treatment irrespective of anything that he might say or do at the time.

This kind of arrangement demonstrates the value of a trusting doctor–patient relationship. Ian is able to transfer decision-making power to Dr McFarlane because he trusts that Dr McFarlane will act in his best interests at a time when, because of his illness, he is not autonomous. Ian's long-term autonomy is protected; his autonomous decision, made when he is well, is to be treated for his illness. Handing over power is a way of protecting his long-term interests. Dr McFarlane is able to intervene earlier in the illness than would otherwise be possible, and to use the directive to override any illness-fuelled resistance from Ian.

This example used a formal mechanism for transferring decision-making power from the patient to the GP; however, less formal examples are common in practice. Patients who are usually thoughtful and decisive may want their GP to make decisions about treatment when they are acutely unwell. For example, a woman who has made informed decisions about contraception and screening may ask the GP to do whatever he or she thinks necessary when she is febrile and vomiting with pyelonephritis. Taking control in this way does not infringe the autonomy of the patient, because it is at the request of the patient.

Treating without consent

Sometimes it is not possible to inform a patient about their illness and proposed management, or to seek consent from them. The patient may be unconscious, incompetent due to a psychiatric illness or mental disability, or have limited understanding, such as in the case of a child. Emergency treatment may be required, for example, to prevent a suicide. If treatment is given without consent, this is known as non-voluntary treatment (see Box 8.3). Such treatment should be based upon what the patient would have wanted for him or herself, if this is known, or, failing this, be in the best interests of the patient. In general, treatment should be aimed at minimizing harm and restoring the patient's health as far as possible. Interventions should be limited to the least invasive consistent with those goals. If possible, definitive or irreversible treatment should be deferred until the patient regains (or in the case of a child, reaches) competence.

Box 8.3 Treating without consent

Non-voluntary treatment occurs when the patient is unable either to give or withhold consent because they:

♦ are unconscious;

♦ are a minor; or

♦ lack capacity to make the relevant decision.

Involuntary treatment is given despite consent being expressly withheld by patient, usually under the authority of mental health legislation.

In life threatening emergencies the situation is usually straightforward: unless the GP has any reason to believe that the patient would not want to be treated in these circumstances, it is ethically required and legally acceptable to provide emergency treatment, aimed at saving the person's life and returning them as soon as possible to a conscious state.

For patients who lack capacity, there are three approaches to making decisions about their treatment. The first, and most autonomy-respecting, is to follow the wishes of the patient as expressed through some form of advance directive. The second is to use substituted judgment; that is, for a relative, carer or legal guardian to work out what the patient him or herself would have wanted under the circumstances. The third approach is to use a best interests standard. Who should judge if involuntary or non-voluntary treatment is in the patient's best interests? Medical practitioners play a significant role in saying whether or not a medical treatment is in the interests of a patient, but any assessment of interests should include information from friends and relatives, and take into account the patient's known values and any previously expressed wishes.

All of these approaches are reflected in law in different jurisdictions. For example, in various states and territories in Australia, patients can complete legally binding advance directives, appoint substitute decision-makers or guardians, be subject to appointment of a guardian by the courts, or have their relatives or carers act informally to make decisions on their behalf. In Scotland, the Adults with Incapacity Act (2002) provides for the appointment of welfare guardians or attorneys with the power to consent to treatment on behalf of the nominated person. In England, the Mental Capacity Act (2005) allows appointment of a donee who has lasting powers of attorney and can consent to medical treatment. Both the Scottish and English Acts use variations of the best interests standard to judge whether or not an intervention should be permitted.

Adults who are incompetent due to mental illness may be admitted to hospital as involuntary patients either as an emergency, for assessment, or for treatment under relevant mental health legislation across a wide range of jurisdictions. The intent behind such legislation is to limit involuntary admission to those who are not competent, by virtue of their mental disorder, to make autonomous decisions (Mason and Laurie 2006). Patients with psychiatric illness can only be given compulsory treatment for their psychiatric illness, not for any concomitant physical illness. This recognizes the fact that, even though a patient may be incompetent for some decisions, this does not mean that they are incompetent for all decisions.

A final group of patients who might require treatment without consent are children. Parents are able to refuse or consent to treatment for their children when that child is not considered competent. If the child is considered competent by the doctor, in terms of being able to understand the proposed treatment, alternatives and consequences, then the child has the right to consent to treatment, irrespective of the views of the parents. (Treatment of children and assessing their competence are fully discussed in Chapter 10.)

External limits on autonomy

Much of our discussion in this chapter has focused on autonomy as a personal capacity or condition for decisions and actions. This approach ignores the wider social context and the ways that choices are framed and directed by external forces. First of all, autonomous choices may be limited by the circumstances of the patient. A patient may prefer physiotherapy to a steroid injection for a shoulder problem, but it may be impossible for them to attend a series of physiotherapy sessions due to childcare responsibilities or difficulties in taking time off from work. A treatment may be too expensive or travelling to the place where it is provided may be too difficult. Public resources may be limited, so that a patient's preferred choice of treatment is not available, either at all or in their area. Patients have many different factors to consider when making decisions, so that personal circumstances can have the effect of directing or limiting choices (Rogers 1999; Jepson *et al.* 2007). These can include the attitudes and beliefs of families and friends, and the kind of opportunities that are available in particular social settings, as well as more concrete factors like access and cost.

The range of options available for the treatment of any problem has been influenced and shaped by circumstances beyond the control of either patient or GP (Rogers 2002). The evidence-based guidelines that are used commonly in clinical practice rely upon research programmes to provide the evidence, but the research agenda is driven by a multitude of interests, reflecting professional and commercial interests rather than those of patients. This means that the range of options open to the patient may not include those that she would prefer (Sherwin 1992). The patient may be presented with a choice between pharmacological or surgical treatment for a problem and be free to choose between those options. However, an alternative approach to treatment–for example, by dietary manipulation, meditation or exercise–may not be offered as an option due to a lack of high-quality information about such options.

At a wider level, people's desires and choices are shaped by the society in which they live, so that, although apparently free to make choices, our ideas about many issues, which feel like our own ideas, reflect widely held values in our society. For example, a woman may be apparently free to accept or reject ante-natal screening or cosmetic surgery, but if the prevailing social norms are to do everything possible to have a perfect baby or a particular physical appearance, we may question the sense in which decisions about these matters are autonomous (Sherwin 1992).

Autonomy and responsibility

In this chapter we have outlined an account of patient autonomy and emphasized the importance of providing information and avoiding manipulation or coercion of patients. What are the implications of this account for responsibility within the consultation? Must patients, to be autonomous, make their own decisions at all times? Who is then responsible for medical care?

First of all it is important to make the distinction between being well-informed and making choices. Respect for patient autonomy requires that GPs provide patients with enough information so that they can understand what is wrong and what might be done about it, unless the patient has clearly indicated that they prefer not to have this information. The responsibility for this lies with GPs. Patients indicate a strong desire for information about their medical problems but this does not always translate directly into a preference for decision-making (Flynn *et al.* 2006). Many patients prefer their doctors to make decisions (Bradley *et al.* 1996) or to share in the process (Deber *et al.* 2007; Murray *et al.* 2007). In general, it is a minority of patients who prefer to make their own decisions alone, although this may change over time as patient expectations change. This leaves much responsibility and control over decision-making with doctors, but in a non-coercive way, as this is with permission from patients. However, this permission cannot be assumed but requires constant checking to make sure that this patient, in this consultation, prefers to take medical advice rather than make their own decision. Much of the time patients agree with medical advice, so that a decision about management emerges from the consultation rather than taking the form of a formal and discrete decision.

Does this leave patients with little responsibility within the doctor–patient relationship? This topic is explored more fully in Chapter 6, but it is worth repeating here that, although patients do have responsibilities, the greater responsibilities lie with the doctor. This can create problems; for example, in determining who is responsible for ensuring that patients receive results from investigations.

Case 8.7

Matthew Slyth came to see Dr Carter with abdominal pain. After taking a history and examination, Dr Carter referred Matthew for gastroscopy,

Case 8.7 *(continued)*

with clear instructions to telephone for the results if he had not heard from the Hackney Road Practice within ten days. In the meantime, Dr Carter went on annual leave. The gastroscopy result came back to the practice, and, in Dr Carter's absence, was given to Dr Chu, who entered the result onto the computer. The report was then filed in Matthew's notes. Dr Carter did his paperwork upon his return from holiday but, as the report did not appear there, forgot about it. Matthew did not telephone for his results at any stage. One year later, Matthew presented with melena from an untreated gastric ulcer, which had been identified by the gastroscopy. He made a formal complaint on the grounds that he had not been given the gastroscopy result.

Transmitting results to patients can be fraught with pitfalls. Posting results or telephoning patients may breach confidentiality, but leaving patients to follow-up may have disastrous consequences, as in Case 8.7. Did the patient in this case have a responsibility to ring for his results? If this is the arrangement agreed between GP and patient, then surely he had a moral responsibility to do so (although the legal responsibility lies with the doctor). If a patient does not ring for results, the GP is left wondering if this is because he or she does not want them, which may be an autonomous refusal of information, or merely due to a slip of memory. Given the fallibility of human memory and the difficulty of eliminating all administrative mistakes from practice, joint responsibility is probably the safest method.

Conclusion

In this chapter we have looked at the important ethical duty that doctors have to respect the autonomy of patients. This duty requires GPs to support patients in making voluntary informed decisions. We have discussed competence, understanding and voluntariness in relation to autonomy and informed consent, and looked at the situation for patients who are not able to give consent. Difficult issues concerning autonomy arise in relation to patients who are incompetent, or who are unable to act autonomously for other reasons. Sometimes the constraints on patient autonomy are external, arising from the circumstances in which people live. Finally we have looked at responsibility for medical decisions.

References

Bradley J, Zia M and Hamilton N (1996). Patient preferences for control in medical decision-making: a scenario-based approach. *Family Medicine* **28**(7), 496–501.

Buchanan A (2004). Mental capacity, legal competence and consent to treatment. *Journal of the Royal Society of Medicine* **97**, 415–420.

Cassileth B, Zupkis R, Sutton-Smith K and March V (1980). Informed consent, why are its goals imperfectly realised? *New England Journal of Medicine*, **302**(16), 896–900.

Charles C, Gafni A and Whelan T (1997). Shared decision-making in the medical encounter, what does it mean? (Or it takes at least two to tango) *Social Science and Medicine* **44**(5), 681–692.

Christie R and Hoffmaster B (1986). *Ethical issues in family medicine.* Oxford University Press, New York.

Cialdini R, Cacioppo J, Bassett R, Miller J (1978). Low-ball procedure for producing compliance, commitment then cost. *Journal of Personality and Social Psychology* **36**(5), 463–476.

Cox K (2001). Informed consent and decision-making, patients' experiences of the process of recruitment to phases I and II anti-cancer drug trials. *Patient education and Counseling* **46**, 31–38.

Deber R, Kraetschmer N, Urowitz S and Sharpe N (2007). Do people want to be autonomous patients? Preferred roles in treatment decision-making in several patient populations. *Health Expectations* **10**(3), 248–258.

Derse AR (2005). What part of 'No' don't you understand? *The Mount Sinai Journal of Medicine* **72**(4), 221–227.

Downie R and Calman K (1994). *Healthy respect, ethics in health care* (2nd edn). Oxford Medical Publications, Oxford.

Ende J, Kazis L, Ash A and Moskowitz M (1989). Measuring patients' desire for autonomy. *Journal of General Internal Medicine* **4** (Jan/Feb), 23–30.

Faden RR and Beauchamp TL (1986). *A history and theory of informed consent.* Oxford University Press, New York.

Flynn K, Smith M and Freese J (2006). When do older adults turn to the internet for health information? Findings from the Wisconsin Longitudinal Study. *Journal of General Internal Medicine* **21**(12), 1295–1301.

Jepson RG, Hewison J, Thompson A and Weller D (2007). Patient perspectives on information and choice in cancer screening, a qualitative study in the UK. *Social Science and Medicine* **65**(5), 890–99.

Kultgen J (1995). *Autonomy and intervention, parentalism in the caring life.* Oxford University Press, New York.

Mason JK and Laurie GT (2006). *Law and medical ethics* (7th edn). Oxford University Press, Oxford.

McMillan JR and Tan JOA (2004). The discrepancy between the legal definition of capacity and the British Medical Association's guidelines. *Journal of Medical Ethics* **30**, 427–429.

Mill JS (1991). On Liberty in Gray J (ed.) *On liberty and other essays.* Oxford University Press, Oxford, 5–28.

Murray E, Pollack L, White M and Lo B (2007). Clinical decision-making: patients' preferences and experiences. *Patient Education and Counseling* **65**(2), 189–196.

Olver I, Turrell S, Olszewski N and Willson K (1994). The impact of a full disclosure information and consent form on patients receiving standard cytotoxic chemotherapy in Stove K (ed.) *Bioethics 1971–2001* (Proceedings of the Australian Bioethics Association Third National Conference) Adelaide, 186–200.

O'Neill O (2003). Some limits of informed consent. *Journal of Medical Ethics* **29**, 4–7.

Ong L, de Haes J, Hoos A and Lammes F (1995). Doctor–patient communication, a review of the literature. *Social Science and Medicine* **40**(7), 903–918.

Rogers AW (1992). *Textbook of anatomy*. Churchill Livingstone, Edinburgh.

Rogers WA (1999). Beneficence in general practice: an empirical investigation. *Journal of Medical Ethics* **25**(5), 388–393.

Rogers WA (2002). Evidence-based medicine in practice, Limiting or facilitating patient choice? *Health Expectations* **5**, 95–103.

Sherwin S (1992). *No longer patient*. Temple University Press, Philadelphia.

Skene L (2004). *Law and medical practice, rights, duties, claims and defences* (2nd edn). LexisNexis Butterworths, Australia.

Sullivan R, Menapace L and White R (2001). Truth-telling and patient diagnoses. *Journal of Medical Ethics* **27**, 192–197.

Young R (2001). Informed consent and patient autonomy. In Kuhse H and Singer P (ed.) *A Companion to Bioethics*. Blackwell Publishers, Oxford, 441–451.

Chapter 9

Ethical issues at the beginning of life

Introduction

In many ways, consultations to do with pregnancy and childbirth can provide some of the most rewarding moments in general practice. Confirming a highly desired pregnancy for a woman or attending the delivery of a healthy baby are times when GPs are able to share in the happiness of patients, privileged by virtue of being a GP to attend at these occasions, but relieved of the need for any medical action, because all is going well. On the other hand, issues such as abortion and the use of assisted reproductive techniques raise a host of ethical questions. Although GPs do not directly provide these services, they are often involved as the first point of contact, with responsibilities for discussing options with patients and referring onto other services. In this chapter, we look at ethical issues in relation to providing contraception, responding to requests for abortions and for referral to assisted reproductive services, providing antenatal care, and caring for women during labour and delivery.

Contraception

Case 9.1

Farideh Ali, a married 24-year-old woman, comes to see her GP, Dr Fiona McFarlane. Dr McFarlane has known Farideh for several years and she has cared for various members of her family, including Farideh's two children aged 2 and 4 years. Farideh is usually accompanied to consultations by other members of the family (often her husband or mother in law); today she seems quite nervous. Eventually she says that she would like to go on the pill, to make her periods regular. After some discussion, Farideh says that she is anxious to avoid another pregnancy in the near future as she is hoping to do some part-time study, but that her husband would not approve of her using contraception. However, if she has to take medication

Case 9.1 *(continued)*

for her periods, then her husband would accept this. She asks Dr McFarlane for a prescription, and for assurance that she will not reveal her request to anyone from her family.

Access to safe, reliable contraception is necessary for women of all ages to avoid the possible consequences of unwanted pregnancies. Without such access, other important aspects of women's lives, such as education, employment or relationships, can be jeopardized. The majority of consultations for advice and information about contraception are very straightforward; once a women is well-informed about the possible options, she is able to make up her own mind as to which method she prefers. Unlike abortion, contraception raises few ethical concerns for the majority of practitioners. Forms of contraception, such as the morning after pill or intrauterine devices, raise questions as to whether these methods are abortifacient rather than conception-preventing. Some practitioners do have conscientious objections to these methods on the grounds that they are destructive of the fertilized egg. Ethical views about when life begins and the moral importance of early embryos vary considerably; these issues are discussed below. Irrespective of a GP's views about these and other forms of contraception, practitioners who do not wish to provide contraceptive services have a moral and, in most jurisdictions, legal obligation to refer patients to other doctors who are willing to provide these services (British Medical Association 2007).

This case raises several issues. First, Dr McFarlane should talk with Farideh to gain a full understanding of the situation. Is Farideh in a consensual sexual relationship, and what are the obstacles to open use of contraception? Farideh may have limited knowledge about contraception and, therefore, may need some explanations before she is in a position to make an informed decision. Once she understands her options, she is entitled to make her own decision about using a form of contraception that suits her. But what of the perceived need to deceive her husband and perhaps other family members, such as the mother-in-law? Dr McFarlane's obligations are to her patient, Farideh, and part of this obligation includes taking account of her patient's circumstances and how best to provide medical care within these circumstances. If Farideh chooses to deceive her relatives about the reasons for taking medication, that is her decision. Dr McFarlane does not need to be involved in this, because the contents of Farideh's consultation are confidential. It is possible that at the next consultation, Farideh may be accompanied by a relative, in which case Dr McFarlane will have to ask the relative to leave the room for part of the consultation. The alternative would be to lie or support the fiction that the medication is for menstrual regulation rather than contraception.

Case 9.2

Mrs Shettleston comes to see her GP, Dr Grainger, about her daughter Maeve. Maeve is 18 years old and suffers from severe mental retardation and epilepsy. She has been menstruating for 4 years; her periods are heavy and irregular and at times seem to distress Maeve. Recently Maeve has started masturbating, and yesterday Mrs Shettleston found Maeve masturbating in the front garden watched by two teenage boys. Mrs Shettleston would like Dr Grainger to refer Maeve to a gynaecologist for a hysterectomy, to prevent any possible pregnancy and to avoid the problems associated with menstruation. She says that unless Maeve is sterilized, she will have to live in an institution as Mrs Shettleston cannot cope with the possibility of Maeve becoming sexually active.

The non-voluntary sterilization of people with mental disabilities raises a host of ethical issues. While GPs will not usually be involved in the final decision, they are often the first to be involved when a request like this is made. What kind of considerations are important here? The first is to recognize the potential for discrimination against people with mental disabilities. In general, we are on hazardous moral ground when we make broad judgements about the fitness of different kinds of people to be parents. Second, decisions about the care of people with mental disabilities must be grounded in the interests of that person, so that the ensuing actions are for their good. Decisions about procedures such as sterilization should be made on a case-by-case basis, and not rely solely on the fact of the patient having a mental disability. It is important to find out whether menstruation is a significant medical problem for Maeve, in terms of menorrhagia or dysmenorrhoea, and what kind of medical solutions short of hysterectomy are possible. If Maeve's menstruation is more of a problem for Mrs Shettleston in terms of inconvenience or distress, there is the risk of using serious and irreversible medical means to solve what is essentially a social problem.

In general, the least intrusive and most reversible kind of treatment, both for unwanted fertility and menstruation, should be tried. Mrs Shettleston may be unprepared for Maeve's emerging sexuality, so that discussions and advice from those with experience in looking after people with disabilities similar to those of Maeve may help her to cope with the situation in a less drastic way. Maeve's best interests, broadly understood, are the most important consideration and must remain at the heart of any discussion about her medical care. In recognition of the importance of protecting the interests of incompetent patients, and the high value placed upon the right to reproduce, many jurisdictions require legal authorization for sterilization of incompetent patients. The courts in Australia and the UK, for example, distinguish between therapeutic and non-therapeutic (or social) reasons for sterilization: for therapeutic procedures, no court permission is required; but only the courts, and not the parents, may permit non-therapeutic treatments for 'social' reasons rather than the direct treatment of disease (Mason and Laurie 2006; Stewart *et al.* 2008).

Abortion

Should the right to control fertility extend to abortion? Despite being illegal in many parts of the world, abortions are common and widespread, with an estimated 42 million abortions (one in five pregnancies) performed worldwide (Brown 2007). Of these, 20 million are performed illegally, leading to the deaths of an estimated 68,000 women (Grimes *et al.* 2006). For some, these figures make abortion very much an issue of public health, as women's health rapidly improves when abortion is legal, safe and easily accessible (Grimes *et al.* 2006).

In jurisdictions where abortion is legal, the legality is often conditional. The conditions usually relate in the first instance to potential risks to the woman or foetus, further modified by restrictions related to gestational age, counselling requirements, performance in specified premises, examination by one or more doctors, residency requirements or third party permissions. Box 9.1 lists factors that are considered legally relevant to abortion in many countries; the extent to which these factors are determinative depends upon the jurisdiction. For example, in the Australian Capital Territory, abortion has been decriminalized and, as with any other medical treatment, requires only the consent of the woman. In other parts of Australia and the UK, abortion is legal only if certain conditions are met. In England and Wales, the 'social' grounds (section 1(1)(a) of the 1967 Abortion Act) require that two medical practitioners must form the opinion that continuing the pregnancy would involve greater risks to the physical or mental health of the pregnant woman or any existing children than terminating the pregnancy. This is by far the most common reason for abortion, accounting for over 95% of all abortions in England and Wales (Mason and Laurie 2006).

Box 9.1 Factors considered relevant to abortion by legal systems

- Woman's request
- Economic or social reasons
- Foetal disability or impairment
- Pregnancy resulting from rape or incest
- Risk to woman's mental health
- Risk to woman's physical health
- To save woman's life

(Adapted from British Medical Association 2005).

In countries where abortion is legal, there is ongoing debate about the upper limits of gestational age at which abortion should be permitted (British Medical Association 2005; Gornall 2007). Abortions after 24 weeks raise questions about foetal viability; many practitioners feel uncomfortable with aborting a foetus that, in other circumstances, would be offered full neonatal intensive care. The majority of women who seek abortions do so early in their pregnancies, but there are situations in which late abortion is required. These include abortions for foetal abnormality, which may take time to diagnose and confirm, or for an emerging health problem in the woman, creating an ongoing requirement for facilities that can offer this service to women.

The reasoning behind most abortion legislation is consequentialist: abortions can be justified in order to avoid serious harms (greater than any harms of termination) that might follow if the pregnancy continues to full term. This way of looking at abortion recognizes that abortion is a significant moral act, but that it may be outweighed by other serious considerations. Gestational restrictions capture the discomfort that many people feel about late terminations for anything other than grave threats to the health of mother or child. However, the legal approach does not engage with two issues that lie at the heart of abortion debates: the status of the foetus, and the right of women to self-determination.

The central anti-abortion (pro-life) argument is that it is wrong to kill innocent human beings and, as foetuses are innocent human beings, it is wrong to kill foetuses (Marquis 1986). On this view, human life begins at conception and any act that intentionally interferes with the growth of the embryo or foetus is wrong. This rules out all abortions, no matter what the circumstances, and equates abortion with murder. Critics of this view argue that a foetus is morally different from a person and that we should make a distinction between being a (potential) member of the human species and being a person. Persons are characterized by certain capabilities, such as consciousness, the ability to communicate and reason, the capacity for self-directed activity and the presence of self-awareness, and it is the presence of these capacities that confers moral status and guides our behaviour (Warren 1999). Genetic human beings that lack these capacities (for example, anencephalic babies) are not persons in this sense and, it is argued, are not owed the same degree of moral consideration. If we accept that foetuses are potential rather than actual persons, they are owed some moral consideration, but not to the extent of overriding the interests of actual persons, such as pregnant women.

For some feminists, the status of the foetus is irrelevant to the abortion debate as the crucial issue is that of women's rights to self-determination. Even if we accept that a foetus is a person and has a right to life, this should not mean that women are obliged to remain pregnant:

> ... having a right to life does not guarantee having either a right to be given the use of, or a right to be allowed continued use of, another person's body, even if one needs it for life itself.

> (Thomson 1971, p.56)

Without the freedom to end unwanted pregnancies, women may damage their health, be unable to care for existing children and have their opportunities in life significantly reduced. For women who suffer failures of contraception or who are forced to have sex, abortion offers the only way to prevent these harms (Warren 2001) and, as the figures above indicate, lack of access to safe and legal abortion compounds these disadvantages and may risk the woman's life.

Abortion for sex selection raises a separate set of issues. This practice is widespread in countries with a strong preference for sons, but is also in demand by parents who wish to 'balance' their families by ensuring that a future child is of the opposite sex to existing children. The arguments in support of sex selection revolve around the idea of procreative autonomy, defined as 'the liberty to decide when and how to have children according to what parents judge is best' (Savulescu 1999). Other reasons for accepting sex selection are the claimed absence of identified harms to either the child, other members of the family or society. Against this, there are claims that sex should not be significant in deciding whether or not to continue with a pregnancy, as both male and female babies are of equal moral value, and that sex selection tends to harm the interests of women by perpetuating discrimination on the grounds of sex (Rogers *et al.* 2007). The legality of sex selection for social reasons varies according to jurisdiction.

Where abortion is legal, access is usually via medical practitioners, giving them a central role. GPs are well placed to assist women in assessing the risks of abortion or of continuing with the pregnancy, and with offering support following a decision. Some women may prefer not to have information about their abortion in their medical records. As removing information from medical records is problematic, it is worth ensuring that any woman referred for an abortion understands how this will be recorded, and any implications for future treatment if the information is not recorded. Most medical systems can, albeit with some reluctance, treat patients anonymously or under a pseudonym although this may increase the costs to the woman.

GPs whose beliefs prevent them from referring women for abortions are obliged to disclose this to patients and to offer to refer them elsewhere (British Medical Association 2007). The fathers of foetuses do not have any legal rights, either to enforce or prevent the termination of that pregnancy. This position recognizes the importance of personal autonomy and the unacceptability of one person forcing another person to have or not have medical treatment.

Reproductive technologies

New technologies raise new ethical dilemmas, and reproductive technologies are no exception. Is infertility a natural misfortune or a treatable medical condition? Does our culture put undue pressure on both men and women to become parents to genetically related, disability-free children, and does treatment with reproductive technologies make the best use of limited medical resources?

There are many places where the boundary between medical and social problems is blurred; however, infertility is a particularly emotive issue. Becoming a parent is central to many people's social identity and overall life plans, so that when this does not happen as anticipated, the anxiety and grief can be overwhelming. As options for adoption are limited in many countries, reproductive technologies offer some people their only hope of becoming parents. However, adopting a medical approach to infertility commits women to reproductive technologies that may be harmful to their health, such as the hormonal manipulation necessary for egg harvesting and the increased risks of ectopic pregnancies and multiple births. As well as these physical harms, the nature of infertility treatments can be alienating, reducing women to the status of producers of ova and incubators of embryos. There is a danger of exploiting the vulnerability that accompanies the desire to become pregnant.

Most IVF (*in vitro* fertilization) centres have success rates around 20%: the average success rate in the UK for IVF treatment using fresh eggs is around 30% for women aged under 35 years. This rate decreases rapidly with increasing maternal age, to less than 1% for women aged over 44 years (Human Fertilization and Embryology Authority 2008). Given these statistics, many women will undertake treatment that is ultimately unsuccessful; a process that may prolong and exacerbate the hurt of childlessness. There are, however, considerable pressures for people to follow the treatment route, given the premium our society places upon having a genetically related child of one's own, and the paucity of low-technology options, apart from donor insemination with informally acquired semen.

These problems are magnified when we consider the wider implications of reproductive technologies. The existence of a medical solution (albeit fairly unsuccessful) creates its own demand: once a technology is available for those who are desperate to have children, people are at least implicitly encouraged to be desperate, to get access to the technology. The focus on producing individual children reinforces current social arrangements in which people have little access to meaningful relationships with children unless they become parents, and diverts attention away from the plight of other unrelated children (Sherwin 1992).

Other ethical arguments against the use of reproductive technologies claim that they are morally impermissible because they separate the natural process of procreation from intercourse (within marriage) or are seen as 'unnatural'.

On the other hand, many people feel that having children is a fundamental part of human life, and that it is wrong to deny people the chance to try for a family. Having a child is sometimes referred to as a right (see Box 9.2). On this view, reproductive technologies are morally neutral instruments necessary for people to realize profoundly important human goals.

Box 9.2 The right to found a family

Article 16 of the Universal Declaration of Human Rights states that 'Men and women of full age, without any limitation due to race, nationality or religion, have the right to marry and to found a family'.

The right to have children or the 'right to found a family' are often cited as reasons to justify the full range of infertility treatments. However, it is difficult to understand how a right to reproduce might work, in terms of whose duty it might be to ensure that pregnancy occurs. In the common course of events a woman can only become pregnant with the co-operation of a man, but there is no general obligation upon men to make women pregnant.

Box 9.2 The right to found a family (continued)

There is no way of guaranteeing the right to reproduce, as even with the best infertility clinics, successful outcomes are not assured. It is not clear whether this right implies that states have an obligation to provide infertility services and, if so, to what level and with what restrictions, if any.

A more practical way of understanding this right is to think of it a right of non-interference: no-one has the right to prevent men or women from *attempting* to found a family.

As well as providing infertile people with the opportunity to have children, using reproductive technologies may avoid harms such as some genetic diseases, or allow parents greater choice about the children they have.

Given the widespread social acceptance of reproductive technologies, a further set of ethical issues are raised in relation to access to treatment (Ankeny 2008). Initially, access to IVF and other technologies was limited to married heterosexual couples. Access by lesbian couples or single women was denied on the grounds of social rather than medical infertility. These restrictions have been relaxed in many jurisdictions: for example, in the UK the Human Fertilization and Embryology Authority (HFEA) recognizes a duty to deal with patients 'without unfair discrimination, whether direct or indirect, in particular on grounds of gender, marital status, race, religion, age, sexual orientation or disability' (Human Fertilization and Embryology Authority 2007, pp.1–1.2).

On a more practical level, GPs are involved in aspects of infertility care once patients have made the decision to proceed. This can vary from advice and support for women who choose to use artificial insemination from informal sources, through to referral to infertility clinics or care of those involved in a surrogacy arrangement. GPs in the UK may be asked to provide information to fertility clinics (with consent from their patients) that might be relevant to the welfare of any child born as a result of the treatment.

Case 9.3

Mr and Mrs Barnett have been trying to achieve a pregnancy for 18 months, without success. Routine investigations to date have not identified any specific abnormalities in either partner, and they report frequent and satisfying sexual intercourse. They now wish to discuss the possibility of referral for further investigation and treatment at the local fertility centre.

Case 9.3 *(continued)*

After initial assessment at the fertility centre, Dr Carter receives a request for any information that may be relevant in helping the fertility centre to fulfil their obligations in relation to the welfare of any child who may be born as a result of the treatment. The leaflet goes on to explain that Dr Carter is not being asked to speculate on lifestyles or to assess his patients' suitability as parents, but merely to provide factual information, medical or otherwise, that might be relevant to the welfare of any child. The request is accompanied by a consent form signed by both Mr and Mrs Barnett.

Dr Carter knows that Mrs Barnett worked as a prostitute several years ago, and that her partner is aware of this. Dr Carter also knows that Mr Barnett has a child from a previous relationship and that he does not seem to have any contact with this child.

What should Dr Carter say in response to the request for information about the Barnetts? The final decision about whether to offer treatment is in the hands of the treating clinicians; however, information provided by the GP, especially if questioning the welfare of any resulting child, may be very influential. In this situation, it is important that Dr Carter consciously avoids any prejudices he might have–for example, about what kind of people make good mothers or the responsibilities of fathers to their children from previous relationships. The GP's role is to consider if there is anything in either partner's history which might be a *significant* threat to the welfare of any child born as a result of this treatment. In the UK the HFEA legislation changed in 2007 to remove the explicit requirement to consider the need of any child born to have a father in relation to the child's welfare: it now focuses upon any previous convictions related to children or child protection orders; serious violence, health or addiction problems; and any factors that may affect the ability of the prospective parents to care for the child (Human Fertilization and Embryology Authority 2007).

GPs may become aware of informal surrogacy arrangements, especially in countries where surrogacy is not legal. Concerns about surrogacy centre on the potential for women to be exploited by using their bodies for the benefit of others; the use of monetary rewards that may constitute an inducement for financially disadvantaged women to gestate for wealthier couples; and the effect on the ensuing child due to its potentially confusing parentage. On the other hand, surrogacy can be an act of altruism or love by one woman for another, and there are many instances of successful altruistic surrogacy.

For GPs involved in caring for the surrogate and/or the potential parents, the welfare of the pregnant woman should be paramount; however the commissioning mother may also require counselling and support through the process.

In pregnancy

Despite widespread recognition that pregnancy and childbirth are not illnesses, in Western societies the majority of pregnancies receive ever more sophisticated medical antenatal care, and the rate of interventions in childbirth continues to rise. GPs may have little influence once patients are admitted to secondary or tertiary care, but they are often the ones called upon to explain test results or advise on options offered by the hospital. This section looks at some of ethical issues that may be raised by antenatal care.

Antenatal screening in the form of blood tests and ultrasound examinations are a well-established part of antenatal care. However, as the range of tests has widened, a number of ethical problems have become apparent. Some antenatal screening is to detect disease in the mother, such as diabetes, anaemia or various infections. These tests are relatively straightforward, as there are effective and largely acceptable treatments for most of the conditions detected. Other forms of screening are to detect abnormalities in the foetus (Aksoy 2001). The reasoning behind the detection of foetal abnormalities is threefold:

- to inform prospective parents and help them to prepare for the birth of an affected child;
- to instigate treatment, either *in utero* or immediately after birth in a suitable centre;
- to allow termination of pregnancy with an affected foetus (Holt 1996).

In theory, screening provides information so that prospective parents can make informed choices between various options. In reality, very few detected abnormalities are suitable for *in utero* treatment, and the choice is between continuing with the pregnancy and having an affected child, or abortion. Current information indicates that the majority of women with pregnancies affected by disorders such as trisomy 13, 18 or 21, Tay-Sachs, anencephaly, spina bifida, thalassaemia, sickle cell anaemia and sex chromosome abnormality chose to terminate their pregnancies (Wertz and Fletcher 1998). The reasons for choosing termination are complex and relate both to the envisaged future of the child, and also the parent/s self-interest (Korenromp *et al.* 2007). It is not clear where the public would draw the line at the kind of abnormalities for which they would consider termination acceptable. Some research suggests a high level of consumerism, with acceptance of selective termination for conditions such as obesity, short stature, missing two fingers or limited musical talent (Henn 2000); on the other hand, the abortion of a foetus with a cleft palate performed in the UK in 2005 attracted considerable public debate. The media coverage was sparked by an unsuccessful challenge to the legality of the abortion, with the courts finding that the abortion was legally performed on the ground of severe physical or mental disability in the foetus.

The first set of ethical issues raised by antenatal screening are to do with questions about the kinds of lives that are considered worth living, and the implications of offering termination for affected foetuses. By framing the issue as one of choice, there is already an assumption that at least some people would choose not to have an affected foetus, and it is this assumption that raises concerns about eugenics and discrimination against people with disabilities. Eugenics is to do with improving the species or the gene pool, either by controlling who reproduces, or by encouraging or discouraging the reproduction of certain characteristics. Does screening for and offering terminations for conditions such as Down syndrome and spina bifida imply a eugenic policy trying to eliminate these conditions from the population? The accepted view of genetic counselling is that this should be non-directive and aimed towards facilitating the uncoerced choice of the individuals concerned, rather than trying to influence the overall make-up of the population. However, there have been challenges to this view. Firstly, non-directive counselling is almost impossible in these situations, especially when the only 'therapy' on offer is termination. The choices that parents face may be limited by the foreseeable level of resources and support available to assist them in raising a child with a disability; where these are minimal, the decision to terminate may be driven by material considerations. In addition, outcome measures used to assess the effectiveness of genetic counselling include measuring the incidence of genetic diseases, where a decreased incidence in affected live births is taken to be evidence of successful counselling (Chadwick 2002).

What about the concern that antenatal screening and selective termination discriminate against people with disabilities? The argument here is that if a foetus is aborted on the grounds that it would be better not to be born at all than born with the disability, this implies that people living with similar disabilities also have lives that are not worth living. This is an implication that many people find offensive, as it makes a judgement about the value and quality of life of people with disabilities. Disability activists make the point that much of their disability is due to the way that society responds to disability, such as the lack of employment opportunities, barriers in the physical environment and discrimination. For example, a study of 36 young adults with disabilities in Iceland found that the type and quality of support offered over time to them and their families were more important than their diagnoses or degree of severity of their disability in terms of affecting their progress towards independent adulthood (Bjarnasom 2005). The limits caused by lack of social supports were far greater than those imposed by physiological disabilities.

Nevertheless, it is not clear that quality-of-life judgements are the only reasoning that prospective parents use. As well as the welfare of the affected potential child, parents also consider whether or not they will be able to cope with a disabled child in the family, and make comparisons between having this affected child or trying for another pregnancy and an unaffected future child (Gillam 1999; Korenromp *et al.* 2007).

There are concerns that antenatal screening and selective termination are the beginnings of a slippery slope, and that once the door is opened to foetal selection, the quest for perfect children will lead to termination of foetuses with, for example, lower intelligence or the wrong colour eyes. Abortion legislation in countries, including the UK and some states of Australia, contain a foetal disability ground, under which abortion is legal for conditions that might cause a severe handicap, but it can be impossible to predict the degree of handicap, especially for conditions like spina bifida or Down syndrome. More importantly, as we have noted, the consequences of the handicap depend very much upon the social context. With advances in genetics, it is likely that the range of conditions for which screening is offered will increase; we will need informed and extensive public debate to develop ethically responsible ways of responding to this development.

A second set of ethical issues are to do with the process of screening and the benefits and harms to women.

Case 9.4

Mrs Nasser had her first pregnancy confirmed at 9 weeks and was booked at the local hospital for shared care and a GP delivery. At 12 weeks she had a dating ultra sound scan. At 16 weeks, she had blood taken for a number of tests. She was told that there is a risk that her baby has Down syndrome and that she should have more tests. Mrs Nasser comes to see her GP, Dr Chu, concerned about what the test results mean and that she may be advised to have an abortion.

Much of the literature about informed choices in pregnancy and childbirth emphasizes the importance of women receiving information and making well-informed decisions about all aspects of their care, including screening (MIDIRS 2002). There is not, however, always time to explain fully what health professionals take to be routine tests, and it is only when a test is positive that the woman is suddenly faced with the full implications of having been tested. Mrs Nasser may not have been aware that she had had a test for Down syndrome, or what a positive result means. The cut-off points for risk estimates vary between different screening services, and different laboratories have different rates of false-positives and false-negatives. Even with a positive result, the chance of having an affected baby is approximately 1 in 60. Mrs Nasser may choose to decline further investigation, perhaps because she does not want to know whether or not she has an affected foetus or because termination would not be an acceptable alternative. If she goes ahead with diagnostic testing, she faces the 0.5% risk of spontaneous abortion associated with amniocentesis (Kozlowski *et al.* 2008).

Screening is usually assumed to be beneficial, in terms of detecting disease or disease precursor states and offering the chance for therapy. But, as discussed, antenatal screening is a special case as at present there is little effective treatment for the majority of disorders that are diagnosed. (See also Chapter 6 for a discussion of the ethics of preventive care.)

The main reason that women have screening is for reassurance that their baby is healthy (MIDIRS 2002). When screening is negative, and the foetus given a clean bill of health, this can be immensely reassuring, but this degree of relief is unjustified as many abnormalities present at birth are not detected by routine antenatal tests, including one-third of pregnancies affected by Down syndrome (MIDIRS 2002). Explaining these complexities together with the hazards and limitations of screening can be difficult and time-consuming, but it is important that women fully understand the implications of tests that they have. (See Chapter 8 for discussion of the importance of informed consent.)

Apart from issues to do with screening, pregnancy also raises issues to do with the dual interests of mother and foetus. Most pregnant women wish for the best possible outcome for their pregnancy and are prepared to comply with medical advice about lifestyle, diet, sporting activities, alcohol intake and so on. Conflicts between the interests of the mother and those of the foetus are rare, but when they do occur, can be very challenging to deal with.

Case 9.5

Gemma is an 18-year-old patient who is a known intravenous drug user. She presents to the surgery with a 3-month history of amenorrhoea, and

Case 9.5 *(continued)*

testing confirms pregnancy. Gemma wishes to continue with the pregnancy and expresses the hope that being pregnant will help her to break her
habit and make a new start. Dr Grainger takes Gemma on as a shared care
patient but, after the first hospital appointment, the consultant says that
Gemma is a high-risk patient and must receive all of her care from specialist services. Gemma makes no contact with either GP or hospital for several
weeks. When she comes to see Dr Grainger, she says that she has been using
again, and that she does not want to attend the hospital clinic, where she
feels despised and unwelcome.

Dr Grainger knows that Gemma's social supports are insecure and that
there is a high risk of her continuing to use drugs.

Looking after patients with addictions poses many problems; these are magnified in pregnancy when maternal drug addiction or alcohol dependency can
damage the foetus. Acting in the best interests of the foetus might suggest
coercing Gemma into hospital admission or an invasive programme of monitoring to see whether she is complying with advice to remain drug free.
However, there are two reasons why this approach is wrong. First, it is never
right to force a woman to have treatment for the sake of her unborn child. We
do not force parents or any other relatives to undertake medical procedures
(for example, to donate kidneys or marrow) for the sake of their children or
anyone else, therefore it does not seem right to demand that pregnant women
place the interests of their foetus above their own interests. Of course, in many
senses the interests of both mother and foetus would be served by ceasing
drug use, but this does not justify coercing Gemma into treatment. Women
have the right to accept or refuse any medical treatments, regardless of foetal
outcome (Steinbock 2001). The second reason why a coercive approach is
wrong is consequentialist; offering support is far more likely to maintain a
relationship with Gemma and lead to a better outcome than adopting a
punitive attitude (Tong 1999).

Labour and delivery

Ethical issues may arise in relation to labour and delivery. Many women accept
medical advice about their delivery, making their choices within the options
on offer. Problems may arise when a woman wishes to deliver in a place or by a
means that is not considered medically optimal. GPs are less likely to be
involved in requests for elective caesarean sections than requests for home

deliveries, although both raise questions about how to respond to difficult or inappropriate requests. (See also Chapter 7 on inappropriate requests for treatment.) There is a significant difference between asking for a treatment, and refusing one. In general, patients do not have the right to demand treatments that their doctors do not believe are indicated. There is no firm obligation upon obstetricians to perform Caesarean sections in the absence of medical indications, but the debate about Caesarean delivery on maternal request has become quite polarized. Some view Caesareans on request as an expression of maternal autonomy and claim that women have the right to decide how and when they would like to be delivered. This is countered by claims that Caesareans on request over-medicalize the birthing process, misuse resources, increase morbidity and mortality for women and neonates through unnecessary surgery, and represent an unwelcome attitude to vaginal deliveries ('too posh to push'). A recent Cochrane review could not find any good evidence about the effects of planned Caesarean delivery versus planned vaginal delivery on morbidity and mortality in women with no clinical indications for surgery (Lavender *et al.* 2006). High-quality randomized controlled trials on this topic are unlikely, leaving practitioners to make case-by-case decisions with the woman in question, taking into account her circumstances together with the issues that we have raised.

Refusing treatment is a different matter. Competent patients do have the right to refuse treatment, such as a Caesarean section or delivery in a hospital, even if this is against medical advice and puts the foetus or mother or both in serious danger. What are the GP's obligations if a patient wishes to deliver at home against medical advice? First, the GP, or perhaps the midwife, will usually have been aware of the woman's preferences throughout the pregnancy, in the context of an ongoing relationship. This provides opportunities for exploring the reasoning behind the decision and for ensuring that the woman understands fully the implications of her decision, in terms of possible harms or delayed access to tertiary care should this prove necessary. It is unlikely that a woman would make an arbitrary decision to knowingly increase the risks for herself and her baby without good reason, and it is part of her carer's duties to understand her reasons. Similarly, it is quite reasonable for the GP to act as medical advocate for the woman and her baby, explaining any risks openly and honestly, remembering that we tend to overestimate risks. The aim should be to maintain an ongoing relationship of trust, whilst trying to reach an acceptable solution. Threatening withdrawal of services would not be acceptable, unless this was in the context of transferring care to another practitioner willing to support the patient in a home delivery.

If all attempts at negotiation fail, the GP still has a moral obligation to care for the patient. GP support will lead to the best possible outcome in the circumstances, even if those circumstances are not what the GP recommended. It would be wrong to abandon the patient because she has refused medical advice, just as patients who refuse advice in other circumstances (smokers with recurrent chest infections, for example) should not be abandoned. Although the baby-to-be-born does not have a legal claim upon the GP's services, the GP, having provided antenatal care, already has a stake in the baby's welfare. Attending the delivery will protect the baby's welfare more than staying away, and meet the moral duty to care for both mother and baby.

Conclusion

In this chapter we have discussed a range of issue that arise in the fertility care of women and potential parents. Many of the final decisions are beyond the responsibility or control of GPs, but GPs are often well-placed to understand their patients and their requests, and to act as advocates for them. In many practices, midwives are the primary carers for pregnant women, and they are often the ones who have to deal with issues as they arise. However, GPs play a vital role in looking after women's health related to fertility, and in ensuring the quality of the care provided by all members of the health care team in their practice. We hope that the examples and discussion in this chapter will help to clarify some of the relevant considerations.

References

Aksoy S (2001). Antenatal screening and its possible meaning from unborn baby's perspective. *BMC Medical Ethics* 2, 3. Available at http://www.biomedcentral.com/1472–6939/2/3 (accessed 23 April 2008).

Ankeny R (2008). Reproductive ethics: New reproductive technologies, in Heggenhougen K and Quah S (ed.) *International encyclopedia of public health*. Elsevier, Oxford, (in press).

Bjarnason D (2005). Is life worth living if you have a disability? In Jonsdottir I (ed.) *PGD and Embryo Selection*. Report from an international conference on preimplantation genetic diagnosis and embryo selection. Copenhagen, Nordic Council of Ministers, 39–56. Available at http://www.norden.org/pub/velfaerd/social_helse/uk/TN2005591.pdf (accessed 23 April 2008).

British Medical Association (2005). *Abortion time limits, a briefing paper from the British Medical Association*. British Medical Association. Available at http://www.bma.org.uk/ap.nsf/Content/HubReproduction (accessed 23 April 2008).

British Medical Association (2007). *The law and ethics of abortion*. Available at http://www.bma.org.uk/ap.nsf/Content/LawEthicsAbortion2007 (accessed 23 April 2008).

Brown H (2007). Abortion round the world. *British Medical Journal* 335, 1018–1019.

Chadwick RF (2002). What counts as success in genetic counselling? In Fulford KWM, Dickenson DL and Murray TH (ed.) *Healthcare ethics and human values*. Blackwell Publishers Ltd, Oxford, UK, 88–92

Gillam L (1999). Prenatal diagnosis and discrimination against the disabled. *Journal of Medical Ethics* 25, 163–171.

Gornall J (2007). Where do we draw the line? *British Medical Journal* **334**, 285–289.

Grimes D, Benson J, Ganatra B, Grimes DA, Okonofua FE, Romero M, Shah IH and Singh S (2006). Unsafe abortion, the preventable pandemic. *The Lancet* **368**, 1908–1919.

Henn W (2000). Consumerism in prenatal diagnosis, a challenge for ethical guidelines. *Journal of Medical Ethics* **26**, 444–446.

Holt J (1996). Screening and the perfect baby. In Frith L (ed.) *Ethics and midwifery, issues in contemporary practice.* Butterworth-Heinemann, Oxford, 140–155.

Human Fertilization and Embryology Authority (2007). *Code of practice* (7th edn), R 2, section G. 3. Available at http://cop.hfea.gov.uk/cop/ (accessed 23 April 2008).

Human Fertilization and Embryology Authority (2008). *Facts and Figures.* Available at http://www.hfea.gov.uk/en/406.html#Treatment_and_success (accessed 23 April 2008).

Korenromp MJ, Mulder EJH, Page-Christiaens GCML, Van den Bout J and Visser GHA (2007). Maternal decision to terminate pregnancy in case of Down syndrome. *American Journal of Obstetrics & Gynaecology* **196**(2), 1–11.

Kozlowski P, Knippel A and Stressig R (2008). Individual risk of fetal loss following routine second trimester amniocentesis: a controlled study of 20,460 cases. *Ultraschall in der Medizin* **29**, 167–172.

Lavender T, Hofmeyr G, Neilson J, Kingdon C and Gyte G (2006). Caesarean section for non-medical reasons at term. *Cochrane Database of Systematic Reviews* Issue **3**, Art no., CD004660, 1–10.

Marquis D. (1986). Why abortion is immoral. *Journal of Philosophy* **86**, 183–202.

Mason JK and Laurie GT (2006). *Law and Medical Ethics* (7th edn). Oxford University Press, Oxford.

Midwives Information and Resource Centre (2002). *Antenatal screening for congenital abnormalities, helping women to choose; and routine ultrasound scanning in the first half of pregnancy.* Midwives Information and Resource Centre. Available at http://www.info-choice.org/ic/ic.nsf/TheLeaflets?openform (accessed 23 April 2008).

Rogers WA, Ballantyne AJ and Draper H (2007). Is sex-selective abortion morally justified and should it be prohibited? *Bioethics* **21**(9), 520–525.

Savulescu J (1999). Sex selection, the case for. *Medical Journal of Australia* **171**, 373–375.

Sherwin S (1992). *No longer patient.* Temple University Press, Philadelphia.

Steinbock B (2001). Mother-fetus conflict. In Kuhse H and Singer P (ed.) *A companion to bioethics.* Blackwell Publishers Ltd, Oxford, 135–147.

Stewart C, Kerridge I and Parker M (2008). *The Australian medico-legal handbook.* Churchill Livingstone, Sydney.

Thomson J (1971). A defence of abortion. *Philosophy and Public Affairs* **1**, 47–66.

Tong R (1999). Just caring about maternal-fetal relations, the case of cocaine-using pregnant women. In Donchin A and Purdy LM (ed.) *Embodying bioethics, recent feminist advances.* Rowman and Littlefield Publishers Inc., Maryland, US.

Warren MA (1999). On the moral and legal status of abortion. In Beauchamp T and Walters L (ed.) *Contemporary issues in bioethics* (5th edn). Wadsworth Publishing Company.

Warren MA (2001 Abortion. In Kuhse H and Singer P, editors. *A companion to bioethics.* Oxford, Blackwell Publishers Ltd, Belmont CA.

Wertz DC and Fletcher JC (1998). Ethical and social issues in prenatal sex selection, a | survey of geneticists in 37 nations. *Social Science and Medicine* **46**, 255–273.

Chapter 10

Ethical issues in the care of children

Introduction

Caring for children is an important part of the work of most general practices. Children attend for preventive care, such as well-baby checkups and immunizations, as well as for the common acute infections of childhood and, increasingly, chronic illnesses such as asthma, diabetes and obesity. In the majority of cases, both parents and GP agree on the care and treatment for these conditions. When there is disagreement about the best course of action, GPs can find themselves on challenging ethical ground. The doctor–patient relationship between GP and parent may be at stake if the medical view is at odds with parental choices.

Case 10.1

Mrs Carpenter brings her 1-week-old son Ben to see Dr Day in his practice in Wilford, rural South Australia. Ben is Mrs Carpenter's third child; he has a sister aged 2 and a brother, Tom, aged 5 years. Ben was born by normal vaginal delivery in the local hospital. At the consultation, Mrs Carpenter says that she would like Ben to be circumcised. His elder brother was circumcised as a neonate in Adelaide, with no complications. Her husband is also circumcised, and Mrs Carpenter says that Ben will feel 'different' if he is the only male in the family with a foreskin. Dr Day asks about Tom's circumcision and, in particular, about the information provided to Mr and Mrs Carpenter at the time. Dr Day is aware of the international literature and growing consensus against routine neonatal circumcision and, although skilled in the operation, is reluctant to perform it in the absence of medical indications. During the consultation, he describes potential complications of circumcision and gives his view that the operation is unnecessary. Mrs Carpenter remains adamant that she wants Ben to be circumcised and that it is a minor procedure; however, she would like Dr Day to do it otherwise they will need to travel to Adelaide for the operation which will be expensive and inconvenient.

Why do children raise particular ethical issues?

In the scenario above, Ben's medical care is being decided by discussion between his mother and Dr Day. Ben has no say in the matter, for the obvious reason that, as a neonate, he is incapable of participating in the discussion or decision. This is the first reason why the care of children raises particular ethical issues: they are incapable of making autonomous choices (deciding for themselves the best course of action, given their situation and interests). The usual default position is that parents make decisions for their children, and the law in most jurisdictions supports this. There are a number of reasons why parents should be granted decisional powers over their children. The first is that society expects that parents will act in their children's best interests as part of the parenting role, so granting parents power is one way of ensuring that children's interests are protected. Second, we expect there to be at least some shared values within families, so that children's values and beliefs are likely to be similar to those of their parents. The likelihood that decisions made on behalf of children will take account of their values and beliefs is, therefore, increased if decisions are made by parents. Finally, parents are the ones most affected by decisions made about their children, which gives them a moral stake in making those decisions. Parents have legal and moral responsibilities for the physical and mental health of their children, as well as their welfare and moral development (Bridgeman 2006). These responsibilities wane as children mature and become capable of making their own autonomous decisions. We take it for granted that parents love and care for their children and will make decisions about their healthcare that protect their children's health and wellbeing. As we will see in this chapter, difficulties arise when there is a difference of opinion between parents and healthcarers about what is in the child's best interests.

A second reason why the care of children raises particular ethical issues is because children are vulnerable. They are vulnerable in at least two ways. The first relates to their physical and mental immaturity, which leads to an inability to look after their own interests. Children, especially babies and young children, require competent care as they are unable to meet their own basic needs for food, shelter, care and so forth. Without such care, they are at risk of harms such as illness, injury and death. In addition, the consequences of events that happen to children can influence their whole life trajectory. Children who are deprived of adequate nourishment, mental stimulation or emotional care can be affected for life. This makes it imperative to strive for the best possible health and wellbeing during early childhood.

A third related reason why children raise particular ethical issues is known as the right to an open future. This is the ethical view that children should be allowed to grow to maturity with the widest possible range of options available to them. Although children in general lack autonomy, this is transient, as the majority of children will grow into adults who do have their own preferences and interests, and the desire to further these. In order to preserve an open future, parents and others involved in the care of children have a responsibility to ensure, as far as possible, that children reach adulthood with all their options intact. For example, one argument against routine infant circumcision is that doing the operation when the patient is a baby removes the option for personal choice when that boy reaches adulthood. If a boy reaches adulthood uncircumcised, he can choose to remain like that or to be circumcised, but as the operation is not easily reversed, circumcision as an infant has reduced his options.

Requests for circumcision

Circumcision is an operation that raises a number of ethical issues. There are different ways of looking at circumcision: it may be an integral part of the identity of specific faith communities, such as the Jewish or Muslim communities, or it may be a social practice based on family custom or the preferences of one or both parents. For some people, these are seen as two different kinds of reasons. We often accord significant respect to religious views; for example, the right of adult Jehovah's Witnesses to refuse blood transfusions is well recognized both legally and ethically. Should we consider religiously motivated circumcision in the same way? What if there is no formal faith-based motive but, as with Mrs Carpenter, she wants her second son to be circumcised to be like his brother and father? On the other hand, those who oppose circumcision see it as a practice that violates the rights of the child to bodily integrity and self determination (Hinchley 2007). According to this view, male circumcision is a form of child abuse analogous to female genital mutilation.

The initial consideration should be the welfare of the child and his right to bodily integrity. As noted above, young infants are not autonomous; they cannot understand the nature of the proposed procedure, nor consider how this fits with their other interests. Instead, their parents act on their behalf, but this is not as simple as consenting for their own surgery given the need to preserve so far as possible an open future for the child. As well as the immediate complications of circumcision, such as bleeding and infection, and any anaesthetic risks, there are long-term sequelae, such as reduced sensitivity, although these remain debated (Hinchley 2007; Patrick 2007). Proponents of infant circumcision argue that the procedure has few side-effects in competent hands, and confers medical benefits, including reduced incidence in childhood of urinary tract infection and reduced rates of sexually transmitted infections later in life.

Consideration of the potential medical harms may influence those seeking circumcision for family or social reasons, and should be discussed as a matter of course with parents as part of the informed consent process. However, the literature on circumcision remains inconclusive and highly debated, especially with regard to the long-term effects on rates of sexually transmitted infections. In addition, medical reasons are unlikely to be influential for those seeking circumcision as part of a religious faith practice. For this group, issues of cultural respect and identity may outweigh potential medical complications.

Does Dr Day have an obligation to provide infant circumcision to Ben Carpenter? This is not an easy question. He is the family GP and, as a rural practitioner, will have ongoing care of the family as they cannot easily find an alternative doctor. A point blank refusal might jeopardize the therapeutic relationship and his capacity to offer future care. The operation is legal, within his competence and it would be a relatively simple process to ensure that both parents fully understand and consent to the procedure. Against this, it is a non-therapeutic, cosmetic procedure with long-term consequences and performing the operation will use local medical resources. Mrs Carpenter has said that they will go to Adelaide, if necessary, so his refusal will not prevent the operation. In this situation, a detailed discussion of the pros and cons and an explanation by Dr Day of his reasons for not wishing to proceed are necessary. If the parents' wishes remain unchanged, it is up to Dr Day whether or not to proceed but, having been through a thoughtful and respectful process, damage to the future doctor–patient relationship will be minimized. The cost and inconvenience to the parents of going elsewhere for the operation should not influence Dr Day's deliberations.

The situation is slightly different with faith-based requests for circumcisions. If access to medically provided circumcision is denied, parents may seek a community member or layperson to perform the operation, with increased risks to the baby's health. Denial of medical circumcision may also compromise the rights of the family to practise their faith without interference and to determine freely the upbringing of their children. In some communities, religious leaders have entered dialogue about circumcision and reached agreement about ritual procedures or delays until boys are mature enough to make their own decisions. Depending upon the circumstances, GPs may instigate debate on this topic, with assistance from local paediatric staff and community leaders.

Female circumcision is widely recognized as an act of genital mutilation with serious and ongoing harmful effects on girls' and women's health. These harms outweigh any rights to religious freedom of expression or the rights of parents to bring their children up free of interference. Female genital mutilation is illegal in many countries; practitioners in these countries who participate in the practice may face legal and professional sanctions.

Immunization

As we have already discussed, the duty to act in the child's best interests can raise complex issues in which physical benefits or harms are weighed against social or religious benefits, against a background of parental autonomy and protection of the child's rights, including the right to an open future. Immunization is a common practice that has done much to improve the health of children around the world, but it is now a contested issue in child health for some parents, raising some of these issues. When vaccines first became widely available, the threats of infectious diseases were very real, and vaccination conferred significant benefit. As the prevalence of the infectious diseases of childhood has decreased, the apparent benefits of vaccination have diminished, and the risks of side-effects and complications have taken on greater weight for some parents.

Case 10.2

Lucy is an 18-month-old toddler, brought to see Dr Buchan by her father. On this occasion, she has otitis media with an associated upper respiratory tract infection and a cough. Dr Buchan notices that this is Lucy's fifth presentation with similar symptoms in the past 8 months and, on further questioning, elicits the information that Lucy has not received any of the recommended childhood immunizations. Her father says that he and Lucy's mother are against immunization because it reduces the child's natural immunity and response to disease, and because vaccines contain dangerous and toxic substances, such as mercury. They have been taking Lucy to see an alternative practitioner who has been administering homeopathic medicines in order to boost her natural immunity.

This is another case in which parental views and beliefs do not accord with accepted medical practice. Immunization is widely accepted as safe and effective. The governments of most Western countries have recommended immunization schedules for children that are supported by incentives such as payments for reaching certain immunization targets or per capita immunization payments. In parts of the United States, children require vaccination certificates to enter public schooling; in Australia, some child welfare benefits are linked to vaccination, and unvaccinated children may be excluded from state schools if there are cases of vaccine-preventable disease. Immunization confers benefit upon the individual child by protecting him or her against infection. Protection for the community is also an important factor, with herd immunity dependent upon a sufficient percentage of the population being immunized. Herd immunity is important to decrease the overall spread of infectious diseases, and also to protect those individuals who are unable to be vaccinated.

One of the major ethical issues raised by vaccination is how much weight to allocate to the community benefits. In general, we do not accept that it is ethically required to undergo medical procedures for the benefits of others; we do not compel organ donation or the treatment of pregnant women for the sake of their foetus. Herd immunity is a slightly different case in that it is a common good such that the whole community benefits if it is maintained, and realization of this common good requires the cooperation of the whole community. Immunization levels need to be in excess of 80–90% in order to achieve protection for some of the common diseases (Strebel 2004). There is scope for exemption of those who would be put at risk by vaccination but, otherwise, community members who do not cooperate may be seen as 'free-riders'. Free-riders are individuals who benefit from a common good without taking their fair share of the costs (in this case vaccination) of maintaining the good.

Should Dr Buchan charge Lucy's parents with being free-riders and explain the community benefits from vaccination? This is unlikely to be a productive approach. Given Lucy's parents' views about vaccination, careful negotiation is in order. First, it is important to find out her parents' beliefs about vaccination and, where possible, offer factual information and explanation in order to ensure that they are as well-informed as possible. This requires Dr Buchan to have some familiarity with homeopathic remedies and other alternative medicine treatments for immunity. Being respectful and avoiding judgmental attitudes and language will avoid long-term damage to the doctor–patient relationship, whether or not agreement is reached over vaccination. For some parents, supply of good-quality information and a careful discussion about their concerns will lead to a change of view. For others, the values are deeply held and not amenable to change (Goldwater *et al.* 2003). In the latter case, once the GP has explained his point of view and provided information to the parents, the decision about immunization rests with the parents.

Complimentary and alternative treatments

Lucy's case raises broader issues to do with complementary and alternative medications (CAMs). For many medical practitioners, the use of treatments that are expensive and lacking in a credible evidence-base is *prima facie* unethical, and yet we know that many patients consult with alternative health practitioners and consume such treatments. What are the ethical considerations here? First, we need to consider the patient him or herself. Is the alternative treatment dangerous, or taking the place of a recognized and beneficial treatment? If so, the GP has a duty to ensure that the patient understands this and is acting freely if they choose to continue against medical advice. This duty requires the GP to have at least some information about CAMs and to provide this to the patient as necessary for their health-care (Brophy 2003). Like all ethical duties, this has to be balanced with competing duties; it is not reasonable to expect all GPs to be expert in all CAMs. There are, however, common CAM treatments, such as for immunity, and others that are important for the care of specific patients, so GPs need to have some basic information about these in order to care competently for some patients. Lacking sufficient information about relevant CAMs can undermine trust and the patient's ability to give informed consent (Kemper and Cohen 2004).

What if the parents' use of CAMs, in the opinion of the GP, threatens the welfare of the child; for example, by replacing an effective treatment? In Lucy's case, not being vaccinated does not pose an immediate and serious threat to her health. However, if she had bacterial meningitis and her parents wished for her to be treated with homeopathic medicines in place of antibiotics, the stakes would be much higher. Ethically, doctors have a duty to act in the best interests of their paediatric patients, even if this involves overriding the wishes of the parents. The law in most jurisdictions supports this position, and there are various legal methods for overriding parental authority, where there is a serious threat to the child's health and the doctor is unable to reach agreement with the parents.

Obesity

Case 10.3

Luke is a 9-year-old boy, brought to the surgery by his mother Elizabeth DeBristo. Elizabeth would like Dr McFarlane to write a letter to the school to exempt Luke from sporting activities on the grounds that he hates team sports because the other children bully him, and running around causes knee pain. Luke is a quiet boy. Dr McFarlane examines him and then discusses the options with Luke and his mother. Apart from being moderately overweight, Luke's physical examination is normal. Dr McFarlane asks Elizabeth a few questions about the family diet and finds out that Luke has

Case 10.3 *(continued)*

always been a 'picky' eater and that he eats large quantities of snacks and soft drinks throughout the afternoon and evening, but does not have a regular evening meal. He spends most of his free time in front of the computer or television, and does not enjoy any physical activities. Dr McFarlane notes that Ms DeBristo is also moderately overweight.

Childhood overweight and obesity are growing problems in Western society (Baumer 2007; Lavizzo-Mourey 2007). How should Dr McFarlane respond in a case like Luke's, in which there seems to be little parental insight? For Luke, his weight is already causing problems in terms of being teased and bullied at school. His increased weight puts him at risk of future health problems, including heart disease, hypertension, hyperlipidaemia, orthopaedic problems and diabetes (Lavizzo-Mourey 2007). As a 9-year-old, he is largely dependent upon his mother for his food, although from the consultation, it is apparent that Ms DeBristo thinks that Luke is in control of food in the household. Obesity prevention and management raise questions about individual responsibility and the role of environmental and social factors (Hinds 2005; Rogers 2008). The latter, such as control of advertising of foods on children's television and the local physical environment, are beyond the scope of action of GPs, who have to focus largely on treatment of the individual. It is certainly in Luke's best interests to bring attention to his weight and the fact that this is a potentially serious health problem. This may be complicated by his mother's denial of a problem ('We are all big in my family') and perceived lack of control over Luke's diet. As with many other problems, the GP must draw upon her skills in building a relationship with Luke and his mother, and in setting manageable goals for his weight loss. As it is Luke's health at stake, rather than that of an adult, Dr McFarlane would be justified in taking a more directive approach than would be the case with an adult with a similar problem. However, the dangers of obesity, unlike those of meningitis, are not immediately life-threatening, so it would be difficult to justify a heavy-handed approach to overriding the parents' care of Luke On a pragmatic level, directive approaches may be less successful than non-directive approaches; therefore, Luke's best interests may well be served by working within the GP-family relationship.

Children raise particular ethical issues in part because just because they are vulnerable: they are unable to look after themselves or make decisions based upon their own best interests. As we have discussed, parents are usually responsible for their children and, in general, parents are allowed a considerable degree of autonomy in bringing up their children according to their beliefs and values. In some of the cases discussed so far in this chapter, there have been differences between the medical view of the child's best interests and that of the parents, leading to questions about the most ethical course of action. In all of these cases, however, it has been clear that the parents are acting according to their view of the child's best interests, albeit based on values that differ significantly in some cases from those of the GP. What of cases in which it the parents or family members who are responsible for harming children?

Non-accidental injuries

Case 10.4

Sheree is a 3-year-old girl. Her mother, Gemma, is 21 years old and lives with her current partner Dan, who is unemployed. Gemma has a long history of substance dependence and drinks heavily at times, as does Dan. On this occasion, Gemma comes to the surgery for painkillers for her headaches. Dr Grainger notices that Sheree is very withdrawn compared to the last time she saw her, and is not using her right arm. Dr Grainger asks about Sheree's arm, and Gemma replies that she thinks it's okay and that she just fell over. When Dr Grainger examines Sheree, he finds marked tenderness over the distal radius and also over her left humerus, along with several small round bruises on her thighs and a healing burn on her back. He decides to send Sheree to the local emergency department for X-rays, and gives Gemma a referral letter, explaining that they will check to see if she has a fracture that may need a plaster. Once they have left the surgery, Dr Grainger rings the emergency department and tells the senior doctor of his concerns about Sheree's injuries, which he suspects are non-accidental.

All doctors who care for children have a duty to be alert for inflicted injuries, sexual abuse, neglect and other forms of mistreatment. The role of paediatricians as child advocates is well recognised (Kurz *et al.* 2006). This role extends to GPs, as they are most often the first medical practitioners to see children and, as they are based in the community, they have greater opportunities to observe family dynamics over time. If a GP suspects child abuse of any kind, he or she has a strong moral obligation to act to protect the child. This obligation is enforced in law through mandatory reporting requirements in most jurisdictions. Mandatory reporting ensures that a competent authority, such as the police or welfare services, will investigate. The role of the GP as child advocate can cause tension if the GP also cares for other family members, including the suspected perpetrator.

How GPs handle suspected inflicted injuries in the surgery will depend upon a number of issues, including the GP's competence in, and comfort with, raising the issue directly with the parents, the severity of the injuries, the need for emergency treatment, any perceived threat to the safety of the GP and pre-existing relationships. In Sheree's case, the GP fulfilled his moral obligation by referring Sheree for investigation of her musculoskeletal injuries and passing on his suspicion of abuse to the new treating doctor, on the understanding that this doctor would refer to child protection authorities. This course of action may not, however, have fulfilled his legal responsibilities as a mandated reporter. Gemma may have become suspicious about the referral and gone straight home, without taking Sheree to the emergency department. At a minimum, Dr Grainger's obligation to her safety requires that he confirm that Sheree did reach the next stage of medical care; if not, he should alert child protection authorities himself.

Dr Grainger did not raise his suspicions directly with Gemma. This is within his rights, but it may be seen by Gemma as deceptive and also may be a missed opportunity to discuss violence within the home; Sheree may not be the only one with bruises and broken bones. A direct and transparent approach in which the doctor raises his concerns and listens to the parent's response can foster trust. However, the safety of the child should be the paramount consideration, whether or not the GP feels able to directly discuss the provisional diagnosis with the parents.

Sheree's case is stark; there is no question that she requires protection if she is suffering fractures. What of less dramatic cases; for example, that of a child requiring regular anti-epilepsy medication and reviews whose parents do not give the medication or keep appointments, resulting numerous seizures and attendances to hospital, or even cases like Luke in which lack of dietary control will lead to health problems? These cases are more challenging than those of overt abuse. This kind of neglect may be the result of parental inadequacies rather than violent tendencies or intentional harm towards the child. Ethical responses include finding out about the home situation and need for external supports, and acting as an advocate to secure these, where possible. Determining when neglect becomes unacceptable can be quite difficult, in part because there are limited options once a decision is made to remove a child from his or her home. Short-term foster care may not be available, and can be suboptimal. Ideally children are best kept with their parents unless they are in danger (physical or emotional), with appropriate supervision and supports to enable the parents to succeed. However, doctors must be prepared to act on behalf of children who are in danger to avoid consequences including long-term disability and death.

Adolescent consent and confidentiality

Case 10.5

Belinda, who is 15 years old, comes to see Dr Carter because her period is 2 weeks late. Dr Carter has known Belinda for 6 years and also treats other members of her family, including her mother and older sister. This is the first time that Belinda has attended alone. She tells Dr Carter that she has been sexually active for 8 months and that her only sexual partner is 17 years old; they have been in a relationship for 10 months. They usually use condoms for contraception but, a few weeks ago, had unprotected intercourse after a party. Dr Carter performs a pregnancy test, which is positive. A long conversation follows in which the possible options are explored. Belinda feels unable to continue with the pregnancy and asks to be referred for abortion. She also asks whether this can be arranged without her parents finding out. Dr Carter makes the necessary arrangements to meet the requirements for a legal abortion, and then talks with Belinda about consent and confidentiality.

There are a number of issues for Dr Carter to consider here. In Chapter 5 we discussed some of these in relation to keeping secrets in families. Here we focus on the criteria for assessing whether or not children and adolescents are able to give valid consent. The criteria for valid consent are voluntariness, understanding and competence (see Chapter 8). Dr Carter has explored Belinda's reasons for seeking an abortion and whether or not she feels pressured by her boyfriend or the fear of her parents' reaction to an unplanned pregnancy. Based upon their conversation, he is comfortable that Belinda has carefully considered her options and is making her own choice. Valid consent also includes understanding and competence, which are related. As discussed in Chapter 8, assessing a person's competence involves asking whether that person can:

- understand the nature, purpose and possible effects of the proposed treatment;
- comprehend and retain information about the treatment; and
- believe what he or she is told and balance this information with other considerations.

This assessment of competence is for adults. However, competence is not an all-or-nothing phenomenon that appears at age 18 years; as children mature they become more competent and, therefore, more able to participate in, and make their own, medical decisions. In recognition of this, many jurisdictions have a test or standard that can be applied to children in order to determine whether they are competent to make the decision at hand. In the UK this is known as the test for Gillick competence (see Box 10.1); this standard has been accepted in Australia following a High Court decision (Stewart *et al.* 2008). In general, a young person is Gillick competent if the doctor is satisfied that, irrespective of their age, they can fully understand the nature and implications of the proposed treatment. If this is so, then that person is competent to make their own decisions without the permission or knowledge of anyone else, even the parents in the case of adolescents.

In Canada and the US, the standard is known as the 'mature minor', which requires that the minor be mature enough to appreciate the consequences of a decision and to exercise the judgment of an adult.

Box 10.1 Gillick Competence

The law recognizes that children mature at differing rates and, while some children may not be mature enough to make competent decisions about their medical care until they are well over the age of 16, others are capable of making those decisions at a younger age. Once a child is mature enough to make competent decisions, the parents no longer have the right to make decisions for the child, or necessarily to be informed about any medical care the child might have, unless he or she agrees. This level of maturity is known in the UK as Gillick competence, after the ruling in the House of Lord in the case *Gillick v West Norfolk and Wisbech Area Health Authority*. Mrs Gillick mounted a legal challenge to a Department of Health circular, which said that in limited circumstances, doctors could give contraceptive advice to children under the age of 16 without parental consent. The trial judge ruled against Mrs Gillick, saying that a sufficiently mature child who understood the implications could give consent to receive contraceptive services. This verdict was overruled in the Court of Appeal, and then reinstated on further appeal to the House of Lords.

In the ruling, Lord Scarman stated that the parental right to determine whether or not their minor child below the age of 16 will have medical treatment 'terminates if and when the child achieves a sufficient understanding and intelligence to enable him or her to understand fully what is proposed' (in *Gillick v West Norfolk and Wisbech Area Health Authority*, cited in Mason and McCall Smith 1999, p.252).

Although the ruling was about giving consent for contraceptive services, the ruling covers all treatment for children under the age of 16 in the UK; that is, Gillick competent children under 16 years of age have the right to consent to any medical treatment. It is up to the treating doctor to decide whether or not a child is Gillick competent in relation to a specific treatment, based upon an assessment of the child's understanding of the nature of the proposed treatment and its implications, and the likely consequences if no treatment is given. The more complex the treatment, the greater the level of understanding required, so that a young child may be able to consent to an injection for a wound to be sutured, but be unable to consent to chemotherapy. For consent to an abortion, the young person would need to be able to demonstrate the same level of understanding of the procedure and its consequences as an adult woman.

There is less clarity about refusals of treatment, especially where there is disagreement between the parents, young person and treating doctors. From an ethical perspective, it seems that if a person is competent to accept a potentially risky or harmful treatment, then they are equally competent to refuse it. The law, however, treats refusals differently, especially where these may lead to the death of the person refusing treatment. In some jurisdictions there are older age requirements for refusals of treatment compared with consent, and at times the courts are called upon to adjudicate if both parents and patient refuse potentially life saving treatment against medical advice.

The right to confidentiality goes hand in hand with the right to consent to medical treatment. If a person is sufficiently mature to make their own medical decisions, then allowing them to do so recognizes their autonomy; that is, their right to be in charge of themselves. Maintaining confidentiality (see Chapter 5) is another part of respecting autonomy: it would make no sense to consider a young person mature enough to make a decision about an abortion, but then breach confidentiality by informing their parents. Such a breach would undermine the young person's capacity to control important parts of her life, including who has access to her private information. Part of the importance of recognizing that maturing adolescents may make their own medical decisions is the assurance of confidentiality that such recognition brings. Emphasizing the confidential nature of consultations in situations like those with Belinda is important; a teenager may be suspicious of adults in general unless specifically reassured that the contents of the consultation will remain private.

The right to confidentiality does not necessarily mean that it is better for Belinda to keep her pregnancy and planned abortion secret. This is an issue worth exploring, as secrecy about health problems can undermine trust and relationships within families. Of course, in an ideal world children would be able to discuss important issues like contraception or unplanned pregnancies with their parents, but when this is not possible, confidentiality must be assured and any decision to disclose remain with the patient.

Conclusion

In this chapter we have discussed some of the ethical issues that arise in relation to the care of children in general practice. Rather than an exclusive relationship solely between patient and doctor, the care of children involves their parents, who have both obligations and rights to make decisions for their children. Parental rights decrease as children mature, and may be overridden if they act against the child's best interests. Doctors must always act in the best interests of the child patient, taking account of the child's vulnerability, her right to care, protection and bodily integrity, and the right to an open future. Older children become increasingly competent and are, therefore, able to participate in, and make, their own decisions, deserving the same respect and confidentiality as adult patients.

References

Baumer JH (2007). Obesity and overweight: its prevention, identification, assessment and management. *Archives of Disease in Childhood Education and Practice* **92**(3), ep92–96.

Bridgeman J (2006). Young people and sexual health: Whose rights? Whose responsibilities? *Medical Law Review* **14**, 418–424.

Brophy E (2003). Does a doctor have a duty to provide information and advice about complementary and alternative medicine? *Journal of Law and Medicine* **10**, 271–278.

Goldwater PN, Braunack-Mayer AJ, Power RG, Henning PH, Gold MS, Donald TG, Jureidini J and Finlay CF (2003). Clinical ethics childhood tetanus in Australia, ethical issues for a should-be-forgotten preventable disease. *Medical Journal of Australia* **178**(4), 175–177.

Hinchley G (2007). Is infant male circumcision an abuse of the rights of the child? Yes. *British Medical Journal* **335**, 1180.

Hinds HL (2005). Pediatric obesity, ethical dilemmas in treatment and prevention. *Journal of Law, Medicine and Ethics* **33**(3), 599–602.

Kemper KJ and Cohen M (2004). Ethics meet complementary and alternative medicine. New light on old principles. *Contemporary Pediatrics* **21**(3), 61–72.

Kurz R, Gill D and Mjones S (2006). Ethical issues in the daily medical care of children. *European Journal of Pediatrics* **165**(2), 83–86.

Lavizzo-Mourey R (2007). Childhood obesity, what it means for physicians. *Journal of the American Medical Association* **298**(8), 920–922.

Mason J and McCall Smith R (1999). Law *and medical ethics* (5th edn). Butterworths, London.

Patrick K (2007). Is infant male circumcision an abuse of the rights of the child? No. *British Medical Journal* **335**, 1181.

Rogers W (2008). Constructing a healthy population, tensions between individual responsibility and state-based beneficence. In Bennett B, Carney T and Karpin I (ed.) *The brave new world of health*. Federation Press, Sydney, 55–72.

Stewart C, Kerridge I and Parker M (2008). *The Australian medico-legal handbook*. Churchill Livingstone, Sydney.

Strebel P (2004). *Epidemiology and global control of measles and rubella*. National Immunization Program, Centres for Disease Control and Prevention. Available at http://www.who.int/vaccine_research/about/gvrf_2004/en/gvrf_2004_strebel.pdf (accessed 23 April 2008).

Chapter 11

Ethical issues at the end of life

Introduction

Case 11.1

Dr Jack Day has looked after Mr Glenn for many years and has an open and trusting relationship with him. Five years ago Mr Glenn was diagnosed with cancer of the prostate gland. Despite an initially positive response to therapy, he now has multiple bone secondaries. His treating oncologist in Adelaide has offered another course of radiotherapy, but Mr Glenn declined this, as the previous course made him feel very unwell, and he would rather not waste time having treatment that is not likely to make much of a difference to the length of his life or go through the dislocation of being treated away from home. Mr Glenn lives with his wife who is well, but who finds it difficult to provide the assistance with dressing and bathing, which Mr Glenn now needs. Dr Day visits Mr Glenn who has a fever and has been vomiting. The probable diagnosis is a urinary tract infection, which will respond to antibiotic treatment. Mr Glenn does not want any more treatments that will make him feel worse or prolong what he believes is the dying process. After discussion about the pros and cons of antibiotic treatment on this occasion, Mr Glenn agrees to have the antibiotics but asks Dr Day not to let him suffer during the rest of the course of his illness. Dr Day assures him that he will provide pain relief and that it will be possible to keep him comfortable. However, Mr Glenn says that he hates being dependant and that once he becomes too weak to feed himself, he would like to end it all and to die with a little dignity. He wants to know if Dr Day can give him an injection when he becomes this weak.

Looking after patients who are terminally ill can be a very rewarding experience in general practice. Dying at home close to friends and relatives, and cared for by familiar nursing and medical staff, is something that many of us would prefer compared with dying in hospital, especially if this is distant from home.

Looking after dying patients allows GPs to use the full range of their clinical, communication and ethical skills as they meet the changing needs of patients. In this scenario, Mr Glenn does not wish to have treatment that he finds burdensome or life-prolonging. Dr Day respects his wishes, tailoring his treatment to meet Mr Glenn's ends. For Mr Glenn, the request for an assisted death may seem a natural extension of the good care that he has received from Dr Day, but for Dr Day, the request raises ethical issues.

We know that requests for help in dying are relatively common in general practice. An early English study found that 64% of GPs had received a request for help in hastening death at some stage during their careers (Ward and Tate 1994). At around the same time in the Netherlands, where euthanasia was first protected from prosecution and later legalized, 97% of GPs had discussed euthanasia or assisted suicide with patients in the previous 5 years, with 73% receiving explicit requests in that period (van der Wal et al. 1992). More recently, an Australian survey found that of doctors who had treated terminally ill patients, 59% had received requests to hasten death by withdrawing treatment, and 43% to hasten death by administering drugs (Neil et al. 2007). European research has similar findings, with requests for terminal sedation, treatment withdrawal or medication to hasten death being requested by 52% of patients during the last 3 months of their lives (Georges et al. 2006).

How do GPs respond to these requests? In the English study, 30% of the GPs who were asked to hasten death complied with this request (Ward and Tate 1994). This is similar to the Australian figure of 35% (Neil et al. 2007), with rates being higher in the Netherlands (Georges et al. 2006).

When GPs are asked about euthanasia and assisted suicide, support for legalization ranges from 40% in Australia and 35% in the UK (Ward and Tate 1994) to 12% in Northern Ireland (McGlade et al. 2000). A study of physicians' (both specialist and general practitioners) attitudes towards medical end-of-life decisions in Europe found that differences in attitudes reflected practices within the countries; so, for example, physicians in the Netherlands and Belgium ranked highest in support for euthanasia, while those in Sweden and Italy were most strongly opposed (Miccinesi et al. 2005). In addition to country being a strong predictor of physician attitudes, the study also found that religious beliefs, type of medical practice and sex of physician were important influences.

The public have also been surveyed about their attitudes towards end-of-life decisions. A review from the US found that roughly one-third of Americans support euthanasia and physician-assisted suicide, irrespective of the circumstances, while another third oppose these practices, also irrespective of the circumstances. The views of the final third vary according to the circumstances, such as terminal illness or unremitting pain (Emanuel 2002). A survey of the

Dutch general public unsurprisingly found much higher rates of support for euthanasia, with 85% indicating their acceptance of euthanasia (Rietjans *et al.* 2006). Despite these differences, there is much common ground in the issues with which patients are concerned at the end of life. These include fear of being a burden to others, concern over loss of autonomy and control over the process of dying, a wish to prevent or avoid unpleasant physical symptoms and loss of dignity, fear of the future, and feelings of hopelessness and depression (Georges *et al.* 2006; Hudson *et al.* 2006; Rietjans *et al.* 2006).

This brief summary highlights some of the ethical issues concerning death and dying. Many people fear dying and turn to doctors for help in shortening the process, either directly through euthanasia or more indirectly through physician-assisted suicide. Doctors may be faced with conflicting ethical imperatives. Respect for the patient's autonomy and compassion for their suffering suggest that the ethical response is to honour these requests. On the other hand, assisting a patient to die undermines respect for human life and ignores injunctions against killing. In this chapter we examine the range of ethical responses to requests for assistance in dying and discuss some of the conflicting ethical values raised by such requests. In the second part of the chapter we look at theoretical frameworks for classifying end-of-life decisions and acts, and discuss some of the arguments for and against the legalization of euthanasia and physician-assisted suicide (PAS).

Ethical responses to requests for assistance in dying

We may be tempted simply to think that requests for euthanasia or PAS should be considered illegitimate medical requests, and that it is a question of personal values whether or not patients and doctors agree with euthanasia. Of course, the situation is far more complex than this. The decision to perform or not perform euthanasia is not a routine part of general practice, but responding to a request from a patient takes place within the same framework of values that informs all general practice.

First of all, the wellbeing of the patient must be considered. It is important to acknowledge the distress that has prompted the call for help, irrespective of the practitioner's views about the acceptability of euthanasia. This can be difficult as few people, GPs or otherwise, welcome discussions about dying. The GP may be the only person with whom the dying patient feels free to voice their distress. Patients may fear upsetting their relatives with open talk of death, or their carers may close off any conversations. Providing support at this time, and accepting the way that the patient feels, are significant responsibilities of the doctor–patient relationship. Voicing a request for assistance in dying takes courage on the part of the patient, and trust that the GP will at least listen and not turn away.

Encouraging patients to discuss their fears and concerns is the first step towards alleviating them. Fear of pain is an important issue, but may be less important than fear of futile or hopeless suffering, loss of dignity, being a burden to others and loss of control or dependency (McGlade *et al.* 2000; Georges *et al.* 2006). Promoting the patient's wellbeing in this situation requires understanding their fears and also understanding how the patient him or herself views these fears in relation to their values: do dependency and loss of control provide the opportunity to receive care from others, or are they experienced as an unwelcome sign of weakness? Once the fears are identified, it is possible to see which of these can be helped by medical care, and to identify treatable causes, such as excess pain or previously unidentified depression. An important part of dying well is coming to terms with one's life and making some sense of it all. Sometimes the distress of the dying is due to psycho-spiritual issues and 'unfinished business' rather than physiological pain.

In terminal illness, it may be difficult to consider the importance of patient autonomy, yet loss of control can be one of the most distressing aspects of illness. Part of Mr Glenn's distress may stem from receiving intimate personal care from his wife, when the established pattern in their relationship has been for him to care for her. He may find personal care from a stranger more acceptable than this role reversal with his wife. There may be no control over the progression of the disease, but autonomy may be respected by offering patients participation in decisions about their care and treatment. Even if the patient does not wish to participate in decisions, keeping him or her fully informed about the process of care is an important way of showing respect.

What if, after acknowledging the distress, and investigating and trying to alleviate the causes, the patient persists in their request for medical assistance with dying (Bascim and Tolle 2000)? What kind of values might inform a GP's response to a request like this? Respect for autonomy requires that patients' competent and informed decisions about medical care should be accorded significant weight. Being autonomous means being able to make significant decisions about one's own life, according to the values that have informed that life. When the period of life remaining is very short, it is surely up to the person concerned to act according to their values, and to be the judge of whether or not the burdens of their life outweigh the benefits. However, there are limits to the interventions that patients may request. While patients have an absolute right to refuse treatment, even life-saving treatment, they do not necessarily have a right to demand specific treatments. There are situations in which it may be justified to withhold interventions requested by patients; for example, when the intervention is not medically indicated or when providing the intervention violates the law. In other situations, complying with legal patient requests may violate the beliefs of the doctor, in which case it may be appropriate to transfer the care of the patient to another practitioner.

Belief in the wrongness of killing runs deep in our society. This is often referred to as the sanctity of life doctrine, implying theological roots. The religious traditions give us a belief in the moral value of life and the notion that life is a gift that humans do not have the right to destroy. Secular traditions place an equally high premium upon the value of human life. The duty not to kill is grounded in the value that we place upon human capacities, such as self-determination, and is recognized in rights theories by the right of individuals to personal liberty and freedom from interference. A utilitarian might argue that killing is wrong because overall the effect of killing upon a society will bring more harm than good. The value that we accord to human life is reinforced by the values of medicine, dating back at least to the Hippocratic injunction to do no harm. The goals of medicine are directed towards protecting and preserving life, rather than intentionally ending it.

Despite these beliefs about the prima facie wrongness of taking life, most societies do make some exceptions. Killing another person in self-defence, or killing opponents in a just war are examples of killing that we usually do not condemn. This suggests that taking life is not always wrong, but that we need to examine the circumstances with care, to think about the motives as well as the outcome of acts that result in a person's death. In terms of responding to a request to end a life, there may be a range of motives that come into play, some of which are morally justified. Compassion for the person suffering is the motive that sits most easily within the framework of medical values. Medical care, in general, aims to relieve suffering and many people think that performing euthanasia can best be understood in the context of providing a release from unbearable suffering. Good palliative care can provide a comfortable death for many people, but there are those who have intolerable symptoms or uncontrolled pain. Withholding medical assistance in dying for these cases condemns the person to extra hours or days of misery, whereas a compassionate response might be to end the suffering. Given the current illegality of euthanasia in many countries, any compassionate acts to end life are supererogatory (above and beyond the call of duty) rather than obligatory. Doctors must relieve suffering to the best of their ability but they are not morally obliged to take on the moral burden of killing a person, or to jeopardize their livelihoods by illegal acts, even if motivated by compassion.

We have already mentioned the importance of respect for patient autonomy at the end of life. Respecting a person's considered and repeated request to die might be another morally defensible motive for euthanasia. Here the justification would lie in the importance of allowing people to be self-determining, and in helping them to reach their goals if they are unable to fulfil these without assistance. Euthanasia activists refer to this as the right to death with dignity, or the right to die. The claim is that, just as we value having control over other aspects of our lives, it is equally, if not more important, also to have control over the circumstances of our deaths. This claim is supported by empirical research showing that control over the dying process is of the utmost importance to those requesting euthanasia (Georges *et al.* 2006).

What are some of the implications if we accept a right to die? The existence of a right implies a correlative duty on the part of others to provide for that right. A recognized right to die would imply a general duty on the medical profession to perform euthanasia as part of (at least some) doctors' activities. Would a duty like this weaken the capacity of doctors to be moral actors? If the right to die relied solely upon a patient expressing a wish to die, the doctor's reasoning as to whether or not euthanasia was an appropriate moral response in this case would become irrelevant, with doctors involved purely for their technical skills, rather than as people with a moral stake in the decision. This could create tension between doctors' duties to respect the wishes of the patient, irrespective of their own views about the person's suffering, and their personal views. In contrast, euthanasia motivated by compassion places some of the responsibility for the decision to act with the doctor, in conjunction with a request for euthanasia from the patient. However, giving doctors sole control over end-of-life decisions is unacceptably paternalistic to those who believe that patients should have the responsibility for deciding to end their lives. In countries where euthanasia is legal, the tensions resolve as, much with abortion services, those who do not wish to be involved in euthanasia pass the care of their patients over to doctors who are comfortable with this end-of-life choice.

What is euthanasia?

In the previous section we used the term 'euthanasia' to refer to the intentional ending of patient's life by medical means, at their request and to avoid suffering; as, for example, would have occurred if Dr Day gave Mr Glenn a lethal injection. This is the way the term is commonly used; a more accurate description of Dr Day's act, should he perform it, would be voluntary active euthanasia. Voluntary euthanasia is distinguished from non-voluntary euthanasia (see Box 11.1).

Box 11.1 Classifications of euthanasia

Voluntary euthanasia

Acting on the competent request of a person to end their life, usually by administration of a lethal drug. The request is generally made in the context of unbearable pain or suffering and/or a terminal illness, and motivated by a belief that, in the circumstances, death is preferable to continued living.

Non-voluntary euthanasia

Acting to end a person's life in the absence of invitation or consent to do so. The person dying is usually incompetent. The doctor or proxy decision-maker believes this is what the person would want and/or that death is in their best interests due to intractable suffering. The decision is generally made in the context of terminal illness, severe disability or permanent brain injury.

These two types of euthanasia, voluntary and non-voluntary, are further classified into active or passive euthanasia. Active euthanasia refers to the intentional administration of a lethal substance, such as an injection of a muscle relaxant, potassium chloride or a lethal (rather than therapeutic) dose of opioid. In active euthanasia, which can be voluntary or non-voluntary, it is the action of the person administering the substance that causes death, irrespective of any underlying disease process.

Passive euthanasia refers to shortening of life by an omission to act. This can cover a sometimes confusing number of options, including:

- not treating a treatable illness; for example, not treating Mr Glenn's infection, if he then died of septicaemia;

- withdrawal of treatment; for example, withdrawing food and fluids from a person with post-coma unresponsiveness; or

- refusals of treatment; for example, a person with motor neurone disease refusing ventilation during a chest infection (Mason and Laurie 2006).

There are significant differences between these 'omissions', as they may be motivated by the patient's wishes (treatment refusal), an assessment of medical futility (treatment withholding/withdrawals) or the view that it is in the patient's best interests to withhold or withdraw treatment. To meet the definition of passive euthanasia, the omission must be intended to cause the death of the patient for the reason that, given the circumstances, death is in the patient's best interests.

Passive euthanasia is widely accepted in many countries, where 'allowing nature to take its course' is both legal and a usual part of medical practice. In contrast, active euthanasia has variable acceptance amongst doctors and the public, and is currently illegal with the exceptions of the Netherlands, Belgium and Luxembourg. But if the intent in both cases is to ensure the death of the patient in order to end their suffering, why do we view the two practices so differently?

The distinction between active and passive euthanasia relies on finding a moral difference between an act and an omission, based upon the claim that we are morally more responsible for the consequences of our actions than we are for consequences that occur if we fail to act. If a patient dies because a doctor gives them a lethal drug, the doctor has killed that person. If a patient dies because a doctor does not give a life-saving drug (or withdraws a life-sustaining treatment), then it is the disease rather than the doctor who has killed the patient. Action implies direct control, whereas with an omission, even though death may be predicted, death is not necessarily ensured by the omission. A person with advanced motor neurone disease may, for example, against expectations, survive a chest infection that has not been treated with antibiotics, to live for a few more days or weeks.

This distinction has proved very appealing both to medicine and to the law:

> The English criminal law … draws a sharp distinction between acts and omissions. If an act resulting in death is done without lawful excuse and with the intent to kill, it is murder. But an omission to act with the same result and with the same intent is in general no offence at all.

(Lord Mustill in *Airdale NHS Trust v Bland*, cited in Mason and Laurie 2006, p.26).

Despite the appeal of allocating responsibility according to act or omission, there are some problems with this way of reasoning. First of all, it may be difficult to decide whether something is an act or an omission. Withholding antibiotics is straightforward: there is inaction on the part of the doctor, an omission to prescribe. Withdrawing treatment is not so straightforward. Turning off a ventilator is classed as an omission (a failure to provide life-support), but turning off a ventilator is an action consistent with our common sense understanding of the term 'act', as is removing a nasogastric tube or an intravenous line.

Turning off a ventilator is a well-accepted example of allowing a person to die, but our thinking may be challenged by the following example comparing two cases of turning off a ventilator. First, a woman with advanced motor neurone disease, who is ventilator-dependant with no prospect of recovery, asks her doctor to switch off the ventilator as she finds her life unbearable. He does so and the woman dies. Under the classification of acts and omissions, the doctor did not kill the patient but allowed her to die–passive euthanasia.

Now imagine the same woman, who has a greedy son, impatient for his inheritance. He comes into her hospital room and switches off the ventilator and the woman dies. When confronted with his act, he says that he did not kill her, but he allowed her to die. Most people would reject his view of events and say that he deliberately killed her: without his action, the woman would have remained alive (Brock 1998). The problem is, however, that the son performed exactly the same physical action as the doctor, so if the son killed the woman, then surely the doctor also killed the woman?

This example helps us to see the moral importance of motive: both the doctor and the son switched off the ventilator with the same intention–for the woman to die, but they had different motives–one morally justifiable and the other self-interested. Despite the clarity of the law in differentiating acts from omissions, the moral world is not so clear. The acts and omissions distinction says nothing about motive and does not always provide a guide to the difference between morally acceptable or unacceptable end-of-life decisions.

A landmark pair of cases in the UK highlighted the paradoxes that arise as a result of the legal acts and omissions distinction (see Box 11.2).

Box 11.2 Similar cases with different outcomes: Ms B and Diane Pretty

Ms B and Diane Pretty both suffered from irreversible neurological diseases. Ms B had bled into her spinal cord and become paralysed and ventilator-dependent. Diane Pretty had motor neurone disease. Both women wanted assistance with dying. Ms B wished to have her ventilator turned off, which would result in her death. Diane Pretty wanted her husband to assist her to commit suicide, as she was no longer capable of physically acting on her own behalf.

The staff looking after Ms B did not agree with her wish to have her ventilator turned off, despite a psychiatric assessment that Ms B was fully competent. Ms B mounted a legal challenge, leading to a ruling by a senior judge that the NHS trust had acted illegally in not respecting her request to have treatment withdrawn. Subsequently Ms B was transferred to the care of a different medical team, her treatment was withdrawn and Ms B died.

Diane Pretty sought legal assurances that her husband would not be prosecuted if he assisted with her death. She took her case to the UK High Court, the House of Lords and the European Court of Human Rights. None of these courts found in her favour, and she died of her motor neurone disease rather than by suicide with assistance from her husband.

Many commentators felt that the moral issues in these cases were very similar: both women were suffering and both women sought assistance with dying (Boyd 2002). The difference between their cases was that one happened to be dependent upon a machine, whereas the other was not. This difference seems to be arbitrary rather than moral: why should the exact nature of the illness dictate whether or not a person can be helped to die? If suffering and a repeated request for help are sufficient in one case, why are these same moral considerations inadequate to ensure help in a similar case?

The doctrine of double effect

The doctrine of double effect offers one way of taking account of the importance of motives when assessing the moral permissibility of actions. This doctrine attempts to distinguish between the intended and the unintended effects of an action, recognizing that sometimes an act with a good effect (such as pain relief) may also have an unintended ill effect (such as hastening death). The effects (both intended and unintended) of actions that meet the conditions of the doctrine are considered by some to be morally acceptable, even if the unintended effects would otherwise not be morally acceptable. There are four parts to the doctrine (see Box 11.3).

Box 11.3 The doctrine of double effect

1. The act itself must be morally permissible.
2. The ill effect, while foreseen, must be unintended.
3. The ill effect must not be disproportionate to the good effect.
4. The ill effect is not the means by which the good effect is achieved.

The doctrine of double effect can be used to justify medical actions that, while intending to relieve suffering, may also hasten death. The classic example is that of administering morphine to a terminally ill person, with the aim of relieving suffering but in the knowledge that the accompanying respiratory depression will hasten death. This fulfils all of the criteria of the doctrine:

1. The administration of morphine for pain relief is a morally permissible action.
2. The morphine is intended to relieve pain rather than cause respiratory depression.

3. The good of relieving pain outweighs the loss of life in a patient who is already dying.

4. The good effect, of relieving pain, is achieved by the action of the morphine rather than by the person dying.

The doctrine rules out active euthanasia, as in euthanasia the act (administering a lethal substance) is impermissible, death is an intended rather than an unintended consequence and the good effect (relief of suffering) is achieved by means of the ill effect (killing the patient).

The medical profession is in general very comfortable with the doctrine of double effect as a way of dealing with medical treatments that simultaneously help the patient but also shorten life. Appeals to double effect provide a way for doctors to answer requests for help in ending a patient's pain or suffering, without performing illegal acts.

In practice, however, it can be difficult to maintain the distinction between intended and unintended effects, and even more difficult to take this as the difference between morally permissible and impermissible killing. It may not be possible to differentiate between the relief of suffering caused by the morphine and the relief caused by death, because the two are so closely linked. Is the doctrine just a way of framing the issue so that we feel (legally and medically) comfortable with this form of active euthanasia? The doctrine of double effect seems to allow euthanasia using certain drugs (such as morphine) but not using other drugs (such as potassium chloride), whose actions may be more predictable or swifter.

Physician-assisted suicide

Physician-assisted suicide shares some common features with euthanasia. Both practises involve doctors acting to help people who wish to die, and both are motivated by a desire to end the suffering of the person requesting assistance. A major difference lies in the process: with euthanasia it is the doctor who administers the lethal substance, whereas with PAS, it is the person him or herself who performs the final lethal act, although the doctor's participation is necessary to obtain the medication. Is this a morally significant difference? On some accounts, this difference is important, because death is clearly the result of the actions of the person involved, making it easier to be confident it is their autonomous choice. But both acts require the participation of doctors and, although with PAS it is the patient who completes the process, the doctor has at least some responsibility for providing the means for the ensuing death.

In many countries, suicide is legal, but assisting suicide remains a criminal offence. If we accept that people have the moral and legal right to end their own lives, than allowing doctors to help them achieve this end with the least possible suffering may seem morally permissible. This view may lie behind the legalization of assisted suicide in places including Oregon, the Netherlands, Luxembourg and Belgium. Oregon has a well-documented decade of experience with PAS, which is legal if a patient suffering from a terminal illness makes a voluntary request for assistance (Quill 2007). The numbers of people choosing PAS in Oregon are small, with a total of 341 assisted deaths reported since 1997. In 2007, 85 prescriptions for lethal medications were written, and of these, 46 patients took the medications, 26 died of their underlying disease and 13 were alive at the end of 2007 (Oregon.gov 2007). Assisting suicide for altruistic reasons has been legal in Switzerland since 1918; assistance is neither limited to nor required legally from physicians (Hurst and Mauron 2003). Under Swiss law, assistance may be offered to any person seeking help, irrespective of their country of residence. In 1998, an organization called Dignitas opened a clinic in Zurich offering assisted suicide. Their services are available to anyone able to travel to Switzerland, including to date some 85 UK residents (Minelli 2007).

Physician-assisted suicide raises some unique ethical challenges (Wolf 2005). The most important of these is how to proceed should the suicide fail. In places where both euthanasia and PAS are legal, a failure in PAS may be followed by active euthanasia, but this option is not available where euthanasia is illegal. The incidence of this problem varies with few failures reported from Switzerland and Oregon, but higher rates in the Netherlands (Emanuel 2002). A second issue is the requirement that the person involved perform the final act, as this means that those with neurological or other disabilities lose the right to suicide by virtue of their disability. If people have a right to assistance with suicide, this should not depend upon a morally irrelevant fact such as lack of motor function or similar.

Table 11.1 lists the different kinds of actions that can end lives, giving examples and possible moral justifications for the actions. As we have discussed, the legal status of these acts varies across jurisdictions, although the moral justifications may be identical.

Practical aspects

Our discussion so far has covered some of the theoretical aspects of end-of-life decisions, trying to clarify the moral considerations that are raised when lives are intentionally ended. In practice, issues are seldom clear, and GPs may be faced with making difficult treatment decisions without the benefit knowing the wishes or the values of the patients they look after.

Table 11.1 Voluntary death and medical aid in dying

Classification	Example	Moral justifications
Suicide	Self-killing by means such as hanging, drug overdose or carbon monoxidepoisoning. No third party involvement.	Right of individuals to self-determination; may be prudent or courageous.
Physician-assisted suicide	Provision of means for patient to kill themselves, such as a prescription for self-poisoning, or insertion of an IV line for patient to inject lethal drugs. Requires medical involvement.	Right of individuals to self-determination; assisting patient to achieve self-determination; compassion for suffering of individual.
Refusal of treatment by competent person	Refusal of antibiotics in advanced malignant disease, or advance directive refusing resuscitation. No third party involvement.	Right of individuals to self-determination; duty of doctors to respect wishes of competent patient.
Withdrawing or withholding life-sustaining treatment from patient	Turning off ventilator in person with stroke, or withholding nutrition from a severely brain damaged patient. May require involvement of others.	Avoidance of burdensome or futile treatment; relief of suffering; best interests of patient to cease treatment; fair use of medical resources.
Voluntary euthanasia (passive)	Withdrawing or withholding treatment at patient's request May require medical involvement.	Right of individuals to self-determination; assisting patient to achieve self-determination; compassion for suffering.
Voluntary euthanasia (active)	Administration of lethal dose of drug with aim of causing immediate death, at patient's request. Requires medical involvement.	Right of individuals to self-determination; assisting patient to achieve self-determination; compassion for suffering.
Non-voluntary euthanasia (person usually incompetent)	Administration of lethal dose of drug in absence of any request; for example, killing severely disabled neonate (active), or withholding/withdrawing of treatment (passive). Requires medical involvement.	Avoidance of burdensome treatment; relief of suffering; best interests of patient to cease treatment
Doctrine of double	Doctor administering drugs with aim of relieving suffering, knowing that side effect may be to hasten death.	Compassion for suffering; death foreseen but unintended.

Case 11.2

Dr Schroeder is doing a locum for a busy urban practice. One evening he is called to the local nursing home to see an 83-year-old woman called Mrs Murray. The nurse who calls Dr Schroeder is from an agency; she has worked at the home on previous occasions but she is not very familiar with the patients. Mrs Murray had a stroke 14 months ago, which left her with a moderate hemiplegia. She is sometimes incontinent and requires help with feeding. Her only daughter lives in France. Tonight Mrs Murray has a high fever and cough. She does not respond to questions from Dr Schroeder but resists undressing. Dr Schroeder examines Mrs Murray and makes a provisional diagnosis of pneumonia. Without treatment it is likely that Mrs Murray will die of her chest infection. Dr Schroeder asks if Mrs Murray has any kind of legal orders about her care or if there have ever been any discussions about treatment decisions in this kind of situation. There is no advance directive, nothing written in Mrs Murray's case notes and the nurse has no idea of Mrs Murray's wishes regarding treatment. Dr Schroeder phones Mrs Murray's daughter in France. There is no reply.

What should Dr Schroeder do? Mrs Murray is not able to say what she wants in this situation, nor is there any indication of what her wishes might be. If she is not treated with antibiotics, she is likely to die. Dr Schroeder's first thought is to act in Mrs Murray's best interests, but this is difficult without any idea about her views of her own interests. Would Mrs Murray see pneumonia as a welcome release from a lonely and disabled life, or would she wish to be treated? Faced with a patient who is unable to make her preferences known, Dr Schroeder considers his patient's medical interests, which would be served by prompt treatment. In reaching his decision, Dr Schroeder considers the benefits and burdens of the treatment: oral antibiotics are not invasive or particularly burdensome, and the benefits are likely to be resolution of the infection with a return to Mrs Murray's previous state of health. In the absence of further relevant information from relatives or those who usually care for Mrs Murray, acting for her medical good is the morally required response. Withholding treatment in this case would be an example of passive non-voluntary euthanasia.

If the circumstances were different, if perhaps Mrs Murray had heart failure and a second stroke, which meant that she was unable to swallow, the balance between the benefits and burdens would change. Treatment would involve insertion of a nasogastric tube or an intravenous line, and there would be less likelihood of recovery to her previous state of health. In these circumstances, initiating a limited trial of treatment or withholding treatment may be morally justified. Situations like these require a careful assessment as to whether or not the patient is in the process of dying, in which case doctors are not morally obliged to initiate or continue treatments that are burdensome and likely only to prolong the dying process, with no benefits to the patient.

Advance directives

What if Dr Schroeder had found an advance directive indicating that Mrs Murray would refuse treatment such as antibiotics for life-threatening illnesses?

Box 11.4 Advance directives

Advance directives or living wills are verbal or written statements expressing a person's wishes about future medical treatment in the event that the person loses the capacity to communicate. They are a mechanism for respecting patient autonomy at a time when the person is no longer able to make decisions and/or communicate their wishes. Usually advance directives describe limits to interventions, such as advance refusal of ventilation or resuscitation, or of antibiotics or parenteral food and fluids, but they may also be used to indicate that a person would like to receive active interventions aimed at prolonging life.

The purpose of advance directives is to enable individuals to participate in decision-making and to control their medical care, at a future time when they are no longer able to communicate. Advance directives can lift the burden of decision-making from relatives and healthcare professionals.

There are some disadvantages of advance directives:

- Difficulties with giving unambiguous instructions covering every possibility, so that it may be impossible to know whether or not the current clinical situation is covered by the instructions.

- Concerns that the intervening illness has caused a shift in the person's identity and their views and wishes, so that the person who made the advance directive in some sense no longer exists. If this is the case, the instructions made by the person prior to illness may no longer be relevant to their post-illness self.

Advance refusals of treatment, if made by competent, well-informed patients, and clearly applicable to the current situation, should be respected. Advance requests for treatment do not carry the same force; doctors are not obliged to provide specific treatments just because a person has requested such treatments, especially if medical opinion is that the treatment is not indicated or is futile.

Apart from the disadvantages listed in the box, the usefulness of advance directives is limited by two further factors. First, there can be practical problems in establishing whether or not a person has made a directive, and then finding it in time to be useful in the decisions at hand. If the advance directive is stored with other important documents in a safe place, it is unlikely to be available to the treating doctors. If the directive is several years old, there may be concern that the person might have changed their mind. Second, the usefulness of advance directives has been limited by an absence of dedicated programmes; such systems seem necessary to ensure that decisions are documented and communicated effectively.

In view of the difficulties involved in writing a detailed and comprehensive directive or living will, attention is now shifting to advance care planning. This involves an open-ended process of communication in which broad aims or goals are described and then revised as clinical circumstances change (Jordens *et al.* 2005). Despite the drawbacks, general practice may be the logical place for people to discuss their wishes about treatment at the end of life, with some record of these being kept with the patient's notes. Discussions that take place with a familiar GP or practice nurse at a time when the patient is relatively well, may be very helpful in informing decisions about future care. Patients' wishes could be reviewed over time (for example, during annual health checks), to make sure that the written information keeps up with any changes in the patient's condition. There are now a number of programmes dedicated to advance care planning, such as the Respecting Patient Choices Program, which provides information and resources for practitioners and patients (Austin Health 2007).

Legalizing euthanasia and assisted suicide

Active euthanasia and assisted suicide are widely illegal, although as Table 11.1 shows, the moral justifications for these practices may be identical to the moral justifications for similar but legal practices, such as passive euthanasia. In this section we discuss the arguments for and against the legalization of active euthanasia and assisted suicide.

The arguments in favour of legalizing active euthanasia draw upon many of the points that we have already discussed such as:

- the right to self-determination and the obligations of doctors to respect and enable autonomous decisions;
- the duty to relieve suffering, even if the only way to achieve this may cause the death of the patient;
- the difficulty of distinguishing between intended, and foreseen but unintended consequences, as per the doctrine of double effect; and

- apparent inconsistencies in the way that the law currently differentiates between people who may be assisted to die on the basis of morally arbitrary distinctions, such as the presence or absence of life-supporting interventions.

In addition to these points, those in favour of legalization argue that the slippery slope of widespread euthanasia in the wake of legalization has not occurred in the Netherlands (Battin *et al.* 2007). Legalizing euthanasia would allow society to recognize the limits of medicine and enable people to discuss their end-of-life wishes more openly and honestly. Finally, they point out that at times, passive euthanasia, such as withdrawing food and fluids, may condemn a dying person to an apparently more prolonged and unpleasant death than administering active euthanasia.

With regard to assisted suicide, the law and society generally accept that people have the right to kill themselves, and that this may be morally justifiable at times, but that it is not legal to assist a suicide. What about people such as Diane Pretty, who want to kill themselves but are not able to because of illness or disability? Does this imply that current laws against assisted suicide discriminates against people who are unable to kill themselves (Doyal and Doyal 2001)?

Those who oppose the legalization of active euthanasia respond to each of these points. We have discussed some of these arguments above, such as the general prohibitions against killing and the problem of framing the discussion in terms of a right to die. There are also a number of consequentialist arguments that refer to the probable harmful effects that might occur following legalization of euthanasia. The slippery slope argument revolves around the concern that once we remove the prohibition against all active killing, there is no logical place to draw a line between acceptable and unacceptable killing. The circumstances in which euthanasia were performed might then expand to include cases that most people would agree are not acceptable. For example, doctors would have no logical grounds for refusing euthanasia to any person who requested it, including those who are not terminally ill. People with chronic illnesses and mental illness would become potential candidates. The very fact that euthanasia was legal might act as a pressure to request euthanasia, especially if the resources to support and care for these people were limited. The other group potentially affected by the slippery slope are those who are not competent: once we accept active involuntary euthanasia for this group, there may be a temptation to shift from considerations of suffering and burdensome treatment to increasing narrow quality of life judgements about the kinds of lives that are worth living.

The legalization of euthanasia might erode trust in doctors, especially amongst the aged and vulnerable, who might feel that any discussions about dying were covert invitations to accept euthanasia. There are also questions about the fallibility of medical diagnoses and the uncertainty of predictions about suffering, that make it difficult for people to make truly informed decisions. Finally, there are concerns that performing euthanasia may have damaging moral and psychological effects upon doctors.

Both those in favour of, and those against, legalizing euthanasia appeal to evidence from the Netherlands to support their cases (van der Heide *et al.* 2007). It is intriguing that despite more than 10 years of experience, opinion remains divided about the effects of making active euthanasia available. There does not seem to be any evidence that the slope is as slippery as feared, although there have been cases of euthanasia performed on people with mental rather than terminal illness, and there may be under-reporting of non-voluntary euthanasia.

Would legalizing assisted suicide avoid some of the pitfalls of active euthanasia? If people who wished to commit suicide could be assisted by another person, including but not limited to doctors, this would remove any necessary connection with the medical profession. For doctors, this might be more acceptable than being the ones nominated to assist with dying. On the other hand, there is evidence to suggest that the public in the UK would prefer euthanasia, rather than assisted suicide, to be available. This may reflect the reluctance on all sides to be involved in actively helping someone to die (Mason and Laurie 2006).

Assisted suicide leaves control over dying with the person concerned, so that there is less likelihood that they might have a last minute change of mind. What about the moral responsibility of those involved? If a GP writes a prescription for a lethal dose of drugs, in response to a request from a patient, is that GP as responsible as she would be performing active euthanasia? Certainly some forms of assisted suicide create a gap between the doctor's actions and the patient's death, leaving the patient as the final moral actor. But what if the patient is, for example, unable to swallow and needs an intravenous drug? In this case the doctor's actions are much closer to the death of the patient, and we can imagine scenarios where there is almost no difference between assisted suicide and active euthanasia.

Conclusion

Assisted dying raises many difficult ethical issues, complicated by various intersections with the law, which leave some practices legal and others illegal. Active euthanasia undoubtedly occurs around the world; whether the incidence of this would change with legalization is unknown. We believe that there can be morally justifiable forms of medically-assisted dying, but as these relate to the context and to the motives of the doctor concerned, it is very hard to develop a framework in which euthanasia 'for the right reasons' would be legal, whilst maintaining the prohibition against other forms of killing. Assisted suicide avoids some of the dilemmas for doctors, but has its own problems, not least of which would be responding to failed assisted suicides.

Irrespective of the legal situation, GPs have a major role to play in providing care to people at the ends of their lives. Compassionate and sensitive medical care can reduce much of the fears and suffering of the dying; over and above the provision of this care at present remains a private matter between GP and patient.

References

Austin Health (2007). *Respecting patient choices program*. Available at http://www.respect-ingpatientchoices.org.au/ (accessed 24 April 2008).

Bascom P and Tolle S (2000). Treatment at the end-of-life. In Sugarman J (ed.) *Ethics in primary care*. McGraw-Hill Health Professions Division, New York.

Battin M, van der Heide A, Ganzini L, van der Wal G and Onwuteaka-Philipsen B (2007). Legal physician-assisted dying in Oregon and the Netherlands: evidence concerning the impact on patients in 'vulnerable' groups. *Journal of Medical Ethics* **33**(10), 591–597.

Boyd K (2002). The law, death and medical ethics. Mrs Pretty and Ms B. *Journal of Medical Ethics* **28**, 211–212.

Brock D (2001). Medical decisions at the end-of-life. In Kuhse H and Singer P (ed.) *A Companion to Bioethics*. Blackwell Publishers, Oxford, 231–241.

Doyal L and Doyal L (2001). Why active euthanasia and physician-assisted suicide should be legalized. *British Medical Journal* **323**, 1079–1080.

Emanuel E (2002). Euthanasia and physician-assisted suicide. *Archives of Internal Medicine* **162**, 142–152.

General Medical Council (2002). *Withholding and withdrawing life-prolonging treatments: good practice in decision-making*. Draft for consideration by Council on 21 May 2002. Available at http://www.gmc-uk.org/ (accessed 23 April 2008).

Georges J-J, Onwuteaka-Philipsen B, van der Heide A, van der Wal G and van der Maas P (2006). Requests to forgo potentially life-prolonging treatment and to hasten death in terminally ill cancer patients: a prospective study. *Journal of Pain and Symptom Management* **31**(2), 100–110.

Hudson P, Kristjanson L, Ashby M, Kelly B, Schofield P, Hudson R, Aranda S, O'Connor M and Street A (2006). Desire for hastened death in patients with advanced disease and the evidence base of clinical guidelines: a systematic review. *Palliative Medicine* **20**, 693–701.

Hurst S and Mauron A (2003) Assisted suicide and euthanasia in Switzerland: allowing a role for non-physicians. *British Medical Journal* **326**, 271–273

Jordens C, Little M, Kerridge I and McPhee J (2005). Ethics in medicine: from advance directives to advance care planning: current legal status, ethical rationales and a new research agenda. *Internal Medicine Journal* **35**, 563–566.

Mason J and Laurie GT (2006). *Law and medical ethics* (7th edn). Oxford University Press, Oxford.

McGlade K, Slaney L, Bunting B and Gallagher A (2000). Voluntary euthanasia in Northern Ireland: general practitioners' beliefs, experiences, and actions. *British Journal of General Practice* **50**, 794–797.

Miccinesi G, Fischer S, Paci E, Onwuteaka-Philipsen B, Cartwright C, van der Heide A, Nilstun T, Norup M and Mortier F, on behalf of the EURELD consortium (2005). Physicians' attitudes towards end-of-life decisions: a comparison between seven countries. *Social Science & Medicine* **60**, 1961–1974.

Minelli L (2007). *DIGNITAS in Switzerland–its philosophy, the legal situation, actual problems, and possibilities for Britons who wish to end their lives.* FRIENDS AT THE END (FATE). London Meeting December 1st, 2007. Available at http://www.dignitas.ch/WeitereTexte/FriendsAtTheEnd.pdf (accessed 24 April 2008).

Neil D, Coady C, Thompson J and Kuhse H (2007). End-of-life decisions in medical practice: a survey of doctors in Victoria (Australia). *Journal of Medical Ethics* **33**, 721–725.

Oregon.gov (2007). *Summary of Oregon's Death with Dignity Act–2007.* Available at http://www.oregon.gov/DHS/ph/pas/docs/year10.pdf (accessed 24 April 2008).

Quill T (2007). Legal regulation of physician-assisted death–the latest report cards. *New England Journal of Medicine* **356**(19), 1911–1913.

Rietjens J, van der Heide A, Onwuteaka-Philipsen B, van der Maas P and van der Wal G (2006). Preferences of the Dutch general public for a good death and associations with attitudes towards end-of-life decision-making. *Palliative Medicine* **20**(7), 685–692.

van der Heide A, Onwuteaka-Philipsen B, Rurup M, Buiting H, van Delden J, Hanssen de Wolf J, Janssen A, Pasman H, Rietjens J, Prins C, Deerenberg I, Gevers J, van der Maas P and van der Wal G (2007). End-of-life practices in the Netherlands under the Euthanasia Act. *New England Journal of Medicine* **356**(19), 1957–1965.

van der Wal G, van Eijk J, Leenen H and Spreeuwenberg C (1992). Euthanasia and assisted suicide. How often is it practised by family doctors in the Netherlands? *Family Practice* **9**, 130–134.

Ward B and Tate P (1994). Attitudes among NHS doctors to requests for euthanasia. *British Medical Journal* **308**, 1332–1334.

Wolf S (2005). Physician-assisted suicide. *Clinics in Geriatric Medicine* **21**, 179–192.

Chapter 12

Role conflicts in general practice

Introduction

Thus far we have focused principally on the ethical issues that arise out of GPs' relationships with patients. Yet many aspects of GPs' work are not undertaken directly with patients. For example, GPs take part in research projects, they attend continuing education events, and they manage the financial and administrative sides of their practices. As they do these things, they develop and maintain relationships with a wide range of individuals and organizations. Such relationships create multiple, and sometimes conflicting, obligations. This chapter explores the ethical issues that can arise because of these multiple obligations.

We will consider these issues through the ethical lens provided by a discussion of conflicts of interest. The chapter reviews the concept of conflict of interest and explores the ways in which such conflicts arise in four specific circumstances–the GP and family responsibilities, relationships with colleagues, inducements to participate in research, and relationships and interactions with pharmaceutical companies.

Conflicts of interest in general practice

We have explored the ethical implications of the GP's role from a number of angles in this book. We have discussed the nature of the doctor–patient relationship and the centrality of trust in that relationship, the importance of confidentiality, the meaning of beneficence and respect for autonomy, and analysed how GPs can manage ethically the competing demands for their time and resources. In all of these discussions, the GP's primary role, and therefore her principal obligation, is the care of patients.

However, while a GP's primary responsibility may lie with patients, this is not his *only* responsibility. As noted above, work in general practice is diverse, involving interactions with a range of individuals and organizations that create a variety of obligations, responsibilities and interests. In addition, most GPs have private and social lives outside their work and these aspects of their lives also generate obligations and expectations. The following list indicates the breadth of roles that GPs fill and the potential for conflict; we will return to these examples later in the chapter.

- In the early stages of an influenza pandemic, Dr Walker would choose to give antivirals to her children, rather than to herself.
- Dr Singh and Dr Schroeder are concerned about patient safety, but also about their own standing in the medical community.
- Dr Chu and his practice receive benefits from their contact with a pharmaceutical company.
- Dr Grainger receives fees for enrolling patients in a clinical trial.
- Dr Carter wants to enjoy his holidays.

The fact that general practitioners are party to a variety of relationships and occupy a number of roles always has the potential to create tension and conflict. Like many other ethical issues in general practice, conflicts of interest are both ubiquitous and unavoidable (Tonelli 2007).

Box 12.1 Conflicts of interest

A conflict of interest arises when one's capacity to fulfil professional obligations seems under threat of interference or compromise because of external interests.

(Adapted from: Thompson 1993; Davis 2001; and Palmer *et al.* 2006).

Each component of this definition is important. First, conflicts of interest arise for people who have specific *professional obligations* or duties towards others. The obvious primary obligation that GPs have is to enhance the health of their patients. However, particularly when they are not directly providing patient care, GPs may have other professional duties. For example, they may supervise students and GP registrars, they may undertake research or they may act as a public health officer. These roles generate different sets of obligations; for example, the obligation to educate students and junior doctors to a high standard, the obligation to conduct rigorous research or the obligation to maintain and submit accurate records for disease surveillance. Some GPs will serve on professional bodies (for example, disciplinary bodies), and these GPs will have obligations to uphold high standards for the profession. The precise nature of these obligations may be debatable and occasionally there will be conflict between the obligations. Nonetheless, what such obligations have in common is that they arise out of the GP's professional roles and they should be the principal consideration in any decision the GP makes.

Box 12.2 Professional obligations and external interests in general practice

Professional obligations for GPs:

- The health of patients.
- The integrity of research.
- The education of students and colleagues.
- High professional standards for general practice.
- Public health practice.

External interests for GPs:

- Financial gain.
- Prestige.
- Public recognition.
- Friendships.

There are also *external interests* such as financial gain, personal prestige, public recognition and friendship bonds that may influence the GP's judgement. Thompson describes these interests as 'secondary' to emphasize that there is nothing morally suspect or illegitimate about these interests in and of themselves. For example, it is quite acceptable for a GP to want to make a reasonable income out of the practice of medicine, and to wish to be respected and valued by her peers.

The third component of the definition, the *threat of interference or compromise* focuses our attention on the fact that conflicts of interest only occur when external interests impact, or appear to impact, on professional judgments. For example, a GP whose desire for financial security leads him to spend his leisure hours playing the stock market has no conflict of interest, unless his investment activities impinge in some way on his professional practice. There is only a conflict of interest when decisions that ought to be shaped by professional obligations, such as a commitment to patients' welfare, appear to be or actually are shaped by external interests, such as financial gain.

The final key word in the definition above is *seems*. Conflicts of interest exist, not only when professional judgment is actually influenced by external interests, but also when it *appears* that an external interest might influence one's professional judgment. This fact focuses our attention on the circumstances in which conflicts arise, rather than on how things actually turn out (Kassirer and Angell 1993). GPs who may benefit financially from enrolling patients in a randomized controlled trial that imposes significant burdens on patients have a conflict of interest regardless of whether they actually do go ahead and enrol patients or not. As Kassirer and Angell suggest, it is 'circumstances [that] determine whether there is a conflict of interest, not the outcome' (1993, p.570).

In some respects, conflicts of interest are unlike other sorts of moral conflict, such as the following conflict between respecting a patient's choice to refuse care and acting in the most beneficent manner toward that patient.

Case 12.1

Mrs Duke, a patient in her late sixties, is an infrequent attender at the Gordon Road practice. One day she presented to Dr McDonald with abdominal distension and anorexia. On examination, Dr McDonald found a large mass and ascites. Dr McDonald thought that the most likely diagnosis was ovarian cancer. She explained this to Mrs Duke and advised that some investigations would help to confirm the diagnosis and then it would be possible to work out what, if any, treatment would be recommended. Mrs Duke refused to have any investigations or to see a specialist for further assessment. She eventually died several months later.

In this scenario, there are two competing priorities–respect for patient autonomy and beneficence. In principle, both are equally important, and the dilemma here is to decide which obligation is greater. Conflicts of interest, however, do not have this equality of priority. Usually, it is clear that professional duty–for example, seeking a patient's best interests–should take precedence, and the problem is how to ensure that external interests do not override the doctor's primary obligation to care for his patient.

One set of interests that we have not mentioned so far is non-financial self-interest. A GP's interest in her own welfare will not always relate to financial issues. It may be, for example, that the personal interests the doctor wishes to promote concern her quality of life (for example, how many sessions she works), her safety (to what extent she exposes herself to infections or to home visits in potentially dangerous situations) or her emotional and psychological wellbeing (how much she takes to heart her patients' burdens). In each of these cases, the GP may be faced with the realisation that her legitimate concern for her own wellbeing may not be in her patients' best interests.

These issues are important, not least because there has been increasing recognition in recent years that some GPs are inclined to pay too little attention to their own wellbeing. While once it may have been acceptable to work 80-hour weeks, never take recreation leave, ignore the needs and wishes of families, and devote oneself totally to medicine, today there is more emphasis on the need for doctors to practise self-care, by ensuring that they take adequate leave, work sensible hours and maintain interests outside of medicine. The moral justifications for 'self-care' can be confusing because we can regard a GP's interest in her own wellbeing either as arising out professional obligations or as an expression of external interests. Doctors' interest in their own welfare can be justified by arguing that the GP who leads a balanced life provides better care for patients than the GP who is chronically overworked. This argument retains the health and care of patients as the primary interest and thus uses professional obligation as the justification for self-care. A second justification for self-care by doctors focuses on the rights that all people have to acceptable working conditions and adequate leisure. In daily life, such conceptual clarity is rare, and the line between self-interest to ensure high standards of care, and self-interest as an end in itself, is often blurred. Deciding how much to give to self and how much to patients will always be a difficult issue.

Why should we be concerned about conflicts of interest?

Conflicts of interest are significant ethically for a number of reasons. First, they can place at risk the relationship of trust between GP and patient. We have explored the concept of trust in detail in Chapter 3; here it is sufficient to note that patients expect that doctors will have their best interests at heart. The fulfilment of that expectation is central to the maintenance of trust. If patients perceive their GP to have divided loyalties–whether or not the GP is actually influenced by external interests–they may question the faith they place in their GP and in the profession generally (Lemmens and Singer 1998).

Second, patients are in a relatively powerless position *vis-à-vis* their medical practitioners; apprehension, weakness and fear, coupled to the knowledge imbalance between doctor and patient, means that patients often need to trust that their doctor will act for them when they are unable to act for themselves (Pellegrino 1987, 1994). In these situations, patients may need to trust their GP's judgement more than they might, say, trust the opinion of the car mechanic who fixes their car. Again, the possibility that GPs may be influenced by interests other than those of their patients can undermine the necessarily trusting relationship between doctor and patient.

Finally, understanding and addressing conflicts of interest are important simply because these types of ethical problems can be among the hardest to recognize. Striking the right balance between family and professional obligations, or between leisure and work, is something most GPs can negotiate fairly successfully without compromising patient care. More troubling are the powerful forces that operate when conflicts are 'systemic': when the conflicts are long-standing, part of institutional practice and involving many clinicians (Tonelli 2007). The way in which general practice is remunerated and relationships with pharmaceutical companies are good examples of situations that can lead to systemic conflicts of interest. It may be difficult for GPs to even recognize these sorts of situations because they are just part of the way in which medicine is practised. In this chapter we explore both routine and more difficult conflicts of interest.

Some specific examples

In this section we provide examples of conflicts of interest. We follow this with a discussion of how to evaluate and resolve conflicts of interest. These examples clearly do not exhaust the range of conflicts GPs may encounter in their work. They are set out here to indicate the types of conflicts GPs face and to provide material for the sections that follow.

The GP and family responsibilities

Some of the most difficult conflicts of interest for GPs arise when the interests of their own families conflict with their professional obligations. Such situations are particularly troublesome because doctors, like anyone else in a personal relationship, have primary obligations to seek the best interests of their families.

Case 12.2

Dr Walker has recently attended a meeting with the local health authority at which GP involvement in pandemic influenza prevention and containment was discussed. The authority has made clear that, in the event of a pandemic, antiviral medication will be provided to GPs who are in contact with patients who may have influenza. The rationale for this is both to protect the GP and to reduce viral transmission in the community.

Dr Walker has two young children and she is concerned about the risk that they may become infected if she is seeing patients with influenza.

> **Case 12.2** *(continued)*
>
> At the meeting she asked about the availability of antivirals for her family. She was told that there will not be sufficient supplies of antivirals for GPs' families to be treated prophylactically.
>
> Dr Walker thinks that she would probably give the antiviral medication to her children before she would take it herself.

There are a number of obligations in this case. First, Dr Walker has an obligation, as a mother, to protect her children. Whether or not that obligation ought to extend to diverting public resources to her family is debatable, but her perspective is certainly understandable. Second, Dr Walker has a professional obligation to provide healthcare for the patients in her practice. While she is probably not obliged to provide personally the care that these patients may need in a pandemic, she does have an obligation to ensure that a basic level of care is provided in the difficult circumstances that may arise during a pandemic. Third, Dr Walker also has obligations to the broader community. The reason that antivirals will be provided for health workers during a pandemic is both to protect the workers and to try to minimize the spread of infection through the community. As a potential agent of transmission, Dr Walker has a duty to try to reduce the risk that those around her will be infected. Finally, Dr Walker has an interest in her own wellbeing, which she seems to discount here in favour of protecting her family. Reconciling competing interests such as these is perhaps one of the most challenging situations for doctors, a fact that has been recognized in recent writing about health worker involvement in epidemics (World Health Organization 2007).

Relationships with colleagues

No GP works in isolation from other doctors and health professionals. It is hardly surprising that relationships with colleagues can be problematic at times. Consider the following examples.

> ## Case 12.3
>
> Dr Singh has worked at the Wilford Practice for several months now. One evening she was in the local hospital in Milton attending a delivery when the senior sister on duty took her aside and mentioned that the doctor on call in casualty that evening had just come in smelling very strongly of alcohol. She was unsure what to do. Dr Singh was not surprised, as it was

Case 12.3 *(continued)*

common knowledge amongst the local medical community that this doctor had a drinking problem.

Dr Singh suggested that they call the medical superintendent in to talk with the doctor and decide whether he was fit to work that evening or not. Unfortunately, when the medical superintendent arrived, he also was drunk and he was unable to make a rational decision about the situation. The medical superintendent then took the sister aside and berated her for her interference. He told her that she should know better than to question the doctor's competence, regardless of whether he'd had any alcohol to drink, and that it was none of her business anyhow.

Dr Singh was appalled by the medical superintendent's actions and decided to take the issue to the next medical staff meeting. At this meeting she was belittled and made to feel that she was young and inexperienced, and that she should not interfere in a situation that required wiser and older heads.

Case 12.4

Dr Schroeder has been working as a locum in a small number of practices for about 6 months. In one practice in particular, he has become very uncomfortable with the way that children with chronic asthma are managed. He has strong views that asthma management in children requires a comprehensive approach that includes home monitoring, asthma diaries and allergy tests. In this practice, doctors do not even take peak flows when the patients come in to see them, relying instead on what appears to Dr Schroeder to be a 'best guess'.

Dr Schroeder only works Saturday mornings in this practice. He acknowledges that his position is short-term and that the patients of the practice are under the long-term care of other GPs. He is reluctant to institute asthma management programmes with the children he sees, because their regular doctors will not follow up the programmes. His solution is to make no changes to the patients' management and just to make some suggestions in the case notes about future management options for them. He couches these suggestions as ideas from another doctor who has just cast their eyes over this particular patient, without necessarily doing much. He does not mention the possibility of different management to the patients at all.

Medical misconduct of the type described in these cases seems to be a particularly difficult issue for doctors to deal with. Some writers suggest that most cases of medical misconduct are ignored by the profession (Rhodes and Cohen 2001). For example, in New Zealand, 'only 45 (17%) of the 267 doctors whose competence was reviewed by the Medical Council of New Zealand between 1996 and 2002 were reported by their colleagues' (Raniga *et al.* 2005). Colleagues are often slow to act because they fear the consequences, both for themselves and for the doctor whose conduct is in question. Doctors may fear being ostracized, threatened or losing their job if they question a colleague's competence. And, they may not be confident that the doctor will actually be helped if his misconduct is reported (Rhodes and Cohen 2001, p.217).

GPs must remember that their primary concern in these situations is the best interests of patients, rather than a secondary interest in the good name of the profession or in their own welfare. The World Medical Association's view here is clear:

> The physician has an obligation to provide his or her patients with competent medical service and to report to the appropriate authorities those physicians who practice unethically and incompetently or who engage in fraud or deception.

> (World Medical Association 2006)

The same message is apparent in the guidance from the General Medical Council in the United Kingdom:

> You must protect patients from risk of harm posed by another colleague's conduct, performance or health. The safety of patients must come first at all times. If you have concerns that a colleague may not be fit to practise, you must take appropriate steps without delay, so that the concerns are investigated and patients protected where necessary. This means you must give an honest explanation of your concerns to an appropriate person from your employing or contracting body, and follow their procedures.

> (General Medical Council 2006a, para. 43)

Even with such clear advice, deciding exactly how to intervene in such situations can be very difficult and a careful evaluation, perhaps with the aid of an experienced colleague, is required. If a GP is concerned about the competence of a colleague, the first step is always to be as sure of the facts as possible. Having collected as much information as possible, the GP should bring their concerns to an appropriate person in a position of authority, such as the medical director, nursing director or chief executive, or the appropriate regulatory body.

For more minor situations of conflict, such as that experienced by Dr Schroeder, it may be possible to address concerns with the doctor personally or within the practice. Despite his temporary status in the practice, Dr Schroeder's primary obligation is to the patients he sees. There is also nothing wrong with telling patients that there is a difference of opinion about how certain conditions should be managed and allowing them to raise these issues with their regular GP (Osgood *et al.* 2000).

Relationships with pharmaceutical companies

The relationship between the pharmaceutical industry and doctors has become a source of considerable tension and controversy. Concerns about the impact of the relationship between drug companies and GPs on patient care arise for a number of reasons (Komesaroff and Kerridge 2002; Alpert 2005). First, there is concern that relations between drug companies and doctors may function to advance commercial interests and doctors' self-interest, rather than patient care or research. Second, there is the possibility that involvement of the pharmaceutical industry in research can lead to biased reporting of research results. Third, public awareness of interactions between drug companies and doctors may undermine the trust that patients have in the medical profession. Finally, there is concern that drug advertising and promotion may influence doctors' prescribing decisions inappropriately.

For GPs the most immediate of these issues is the last one. Many (if not most) doctors believe that they make prescribing decisions based on their clinical experience and the scientific evidence. They ignore, however, the subtle effects of advertising on their prescribing behaviour. In fact, as Blumenthal notes, there is considerable evidence that advertising by drug companies does affect doctors' decision making:

> In a very thorough review of the literature on the effects of interactions with drug companies on physician behaviour, Wazana … found that a wide variety of interactions… were associated with changes in physicians' use of medications. Involved physicians were more likely to request the inclusion of the company's drugs on hospital and health maintenance organization formularies, more likely to prescribe the company's products, and less likely to prescribe generic medications.

> (Blumental 2004, pp.1887–1888)

The interactions that Wazana assessed included the full range of ways in which drug companies and doctors meet each other: direct contact with company representatives, gifts, drug samples, free meals, attendance at events sponsored by drug companies, and support for travel and conference attendance. For example, Chren and Landefeld (1994) found that doctors who received honoraria from drug companies to speak at meetings were 21 times more likely to ask that the companies' products be included in their hospital's formulary. Despite this evidence, most doctors believe that they are not influenced by contact with pharmaceutical companies; ironically, they are not nearly as confident about the independence of their colleagues (Blumenthal 2004).

Pharmaceutical company sponsorship of scientific meetings and continuing medical education activities poses particular difficulties for GPs. Doctors and drug companies both stand to gain from such activities; educational events, particularly, may be expensive to mount and sponsorship can provide a welcome injection of funds. However, there is clear evidence here, as elsewhere, that drug company sponsorship of educational events increases prescriptions of drugs marketed by that company (Komesaroff and Kerridge 2002; Blumenthal 2004; Tonelli 2007).

Those who are against drug advertising, in all its forms, argue that the evidence above leads to the conclusion that drug promotion can result in individual patients receiving treatment that is not warranted. In addition, they point to the high cost of pharmaceuticals and the impact that unnecessary prescribing has on the overall cost of healthcare (Alpert 2005).

Against such evidence of the negative impact of pharmaceutical advertising, many GPs argue that the information provided by drug companies is helpful and that they rely on it to make their own independent assessments (Weber 2001). Even if they accept that support from pharmaceutical companies does have an impact on their prescribing habits, they may argue that the outcome is rarely detrimental to patients. Many patients will actually benefit from having a particular drug prescribed. There is also the argument that some activities sponsored by pharmaceutical companies are worthwhile in their own right, as they provide opportunities for education and exchange of ideas that would otherwise not be available.

Consider, for example, the situation of Dr Chu below.

Case 12.5

With 25% of his patients HIV positive, Dr Chu has developed an interest in HIV medicine, particularly in the management of AIDS in primary care settings. He works with a team of nurses, health visitors, psychologists and social workers with expertise in this area.

Once a month, Dr Chu hosts an HIV case conference in his practice. It is a breakfast meeting attended by staff in the practice and surrounding practices, who have an interest in the care of patients with HIV/AIDS. The breakfast is provided by Links-Howard, a pharmaceutical company that produces a range of drugs used in the treatment of HIV/AIDS. One of the Links-Howard pharmaceutical representatives also attends these meetings.

> **Case 12.5** (continued)
>
> The meetings usually begin informally as the participants eat breakfast together. They then spend about half an hour either discussing general treatment and management issues or one participant will bring a difficult case to the meeting. Dr Chu allows the Links-Howard representative to bring promotional literature and pens to the meeting, and there is also the opportunity to speak to individual doctors at the end of each meeting.
>
> Links-Howard also regularly offers to pay for Dr Chu's attendance at conferences related to HIV/AIDS. About once per year, Dr Chu accepts Links-Howard's invitation, usually to attend a conference in the United States.

Dr Chu probably believes that his contact with Links-Howard in its various forms has little or no impact on his practice. In particular, he may feel that his expertise in HIV medicine allows him to judge impartially the information that the Links-Howard representatives offer him and his colleagues. The empirical evidence set out above can make uncomfortable reading for GPs like Dr Chu, who believe that their own clinical judgment is not influenced by their contact with the pharmaceutical industry.

Dr Chu's most powerful reason for maintaining his contact with Links-Howard is likely to be that he feels the breakfast meetings achieve a great deal of good, with relatively little likelihood of harm. The scientific updates provide an easy way for staff to increase their knowledge and skills and the monthly case conferences allow the practice to review and enhance its quality of care. Dr Chu may also believe that providing breakfast is a simple courtesy to people who are adding an extra activity on to already busy lives.

These arguments for and against accepting gifts, money and sponsorship from drug companies make evaluation of conflict of interest in this arena particularly difficult. A similar set of issues arises for GPs who accept payments for enrolling patients into clinical trials.

Inducements to participate in research

> ## Case 12.6
>
> Mr Shawlands is approached by his GP, Dr Grainger, to take part in a clinical trial. Dr Grainger tells Mr Shawlands that involvement in the trial will mean that his hypertension is monitored carefully for the duration of the trial and he implies that this might not happen otherwise. He also suggests that Mr Shawlands is doing something worthwhile for society if he agrees

Case 12.6 *(continued)*

to take part, just as Dr Grainger's participation is also helping the advancement of science. Mr Shawlands agrees to participate, mainly because he admires Dr Grainger and likes to think they are both helping a good cause.

Mr Shawlands finds his involvement in the trial rather inconvenient, as it involves a number of extra trips to the surgery. Sometimes he needs to take time off work to attend.

About halfway through the trial Mr Shawlands learns from a friend that Dr Grainger is receiving £500 for every patient he enrols in the trial.

There are a number of ethical issues in this case. As with the previous examples, Dr Grainger's primary obligation is to further the best interests of his patients, with or without their participation in any research. The suggestion that participation in the trial will secure regular monitoring of Mr Shaw's blood pressure, which would not otherwise be available, is of concern, suggesting that routine care is not of a high standard or that Dr Grainger is exaggerating the benefits. We might also be concerned about the extent to which Mr Shawlands has given his informed consent to participate in this trial, on the basis of the way Dr Grainger appears to have described the trial to him. Finally, the inconvenience Mr Shawlands is experiencing does not seem trivial and it is important to explore the possibility that Mr Shawlands is actually being harmed by his involvement in the trial.

The ethical concerns expressed above do not address at all the conflict of interest that Dr Grainger has in taking part in this research. In the next section we set out a number of strategies for evaluating such conflicts.

Evaluating conflicts of interest

The problem with conflicts of interest is not that they exist, but the extent to which they engender morally unacceptable conduct. We can evaluate the moral acceptability of a conflict of interest by considering four components of the conflict:

◆ how avoidable the conflict is;

◆ the legitimacy of obligations and interests;

◆ the likelihood that professional judgment will be influenced, or appear to be influenced by secondary interests; and

◆ the seriousness of the impact on professional obligations (Thompson 1993; Goold 2000).

How avoidable is this conflict of interest?

Some conflicts of interest are inevitable. For example, the means through which GPs are paid inevitably generates some conflict of interest, whether GPs are salaried, paid through a capitation scheme or receive fee-for-service payments. Salaried GPs are employees, receiving a payment, usually on a fortnightly or monthly basis, in return for working a specified number of hours per week. Capitation systems reward GPs in the form of payment for each patient registered with their practice. Fee-for-service systems provide a payment for each episode or item of care the GP provides, generally with variations in the payment depending on the type of service provided. In addition to these basic payment mechanisms, some health systems will offer additional target payments to GPs who reach a certain level of service for their patients. For example, many immunization programmes offer a payment to GPs once the proportion of their patient population immunized reaches a particular level.

There is a common sense view that these payment systems subtly shape how GPs practise (Gosden *et al.* 2001). Table 12.1 provides a summary of how payment mechanisms appear to influence practice behaviour. The general pattern is that salaried and capitation systems tend to lead to under-treatment, and fee-for-service and target payments tend to lead to over-treatment. However, there is relatively little empirical evidence to support these contentions. A systematic review of the impact of payment method of behaviour of GPs found that GPs paid on a fee-for-service basis provide more primary care services than GPs who are salaried or receive fees based on a capitation system. It was not clear in this study whether this had an impact on health outcomes for patients.

It is not reasonable to expect that GPs will be completely disinterested in the relationship between their income and their workload. We need to accept that this is a conflict that cannot be avoided completely. What is important is that GPs do not allow concerns about income to shape their practice behaviour in ways that adversely affect their patients.

On the other hand, some conflicts can be avoided. Consider, for example, the following scenarios.

Case 12.8

Dr Singh is covering the practice of a friend, Dr Lomas, who has taken extended leave to visit family overseas. During her 6 weeks covering the practice, Dr Singh sees a number of elderly patients who come in on a monthly basis to have their blood pressure checked. Nearly all of these patients have stable blood pressure and Dr Singh cannot understand why she needs to see them so regularly. For two of the patients, the trip to the surgery is time-consuming and expensive, as they do not drive and need to rely on family or irregular public transport to reach the surgery.

Dr Singh queries the need for these visits with the practice nurse, who suggests that the patients like to chat to Dr Lomas and this is a good enough reason for their attendance at the surgery. She implies that Dr Lomas relies on the fees generated from these patients to prop up his income.

Case 12.9

Every year Dr Carter takes his family on an overseas holiday, often to Australia, where his wife has relatives. He believes that this break is essential to his health and wellbeing. To maximize the time abroad, Dr Carter generally arrives back in the UK on the morning he is due to start work again. He showers at the airport and drives directly to his inner London practice to start work at 9.00 a.m.

Dr Carter's colleagues and staff are beginning to express their annoyance with his behaviour. For the last couple of years, there have been complaints from patients that Dr Carter seems unable to concentrate on their problems during his first days back. Dr Carter, however, insists that he is fine and that he needs every minute of his time away.

On the surface, it appears that Dr Lomas' concern about his income is leading him to provide unnecessary services to patients. He appears to have a conflict of interest between, on the one hand, his professional obligations to his patients and his obligation to society to use health resources wisely and, on the other, his personal interest in his income. Dr Lomas cannot completely remove the conflict, as there will inevitably be some interplay between services provided and income; however, he can reconsider whether his interest in his own wellbeing is disadvantaging his patients and needlessly squandering public resources.

Table 12.1 Summary of potential incentives associated with General Practitioner payment systems (Gosden *et al.* 2001)

Capitation	Salary	Fee-for-service	Target payment
1. Contain costs (personal and financial) and per patient by:	1. Contain personal costs during working hours by:	1. Contain costs (personal and financial) per item of service.	1. Contain costs (personal and financial) of achieving target by:
- Selecting low-risk patients ('cream-skim') (if can refuse patients or fee is not riskadjusted) - Using other services (e.g. referral/ prescription, if not at financial risk). - Providing preventative care. - Pooling risk (e.g. group practice).	- Selecting low-risk patients ('cream-skim') (if can refuse patients) - Using other services. (e.g. referral/ prescription) - Minimizing number of consultations.	2. Induce demand (if marginal cost is less than marginal income) when: - Uncertainty exists about appropriate treatment. - Workload is low. - Supply of GPs is high (income maximizing GPs only). - Fees fall (GPs with target income only).	- Providing target level of care only. - Providing no care if there is a risk of not meeting target.
2. Attract and retain patients by: Price or non-price (quality of care) competition		3. Increase quantity of care are as long as fee is greater than marginal cost (income maximising GPs only) by: - Attracting patients. - Working longer hours. - Concentrate on profitable fee-paying services only.	

Dr Carter has a conflict of interest between his professional obligations to his patients and his colleagues, and his external interest in a relaxing and satisfying holiday. However, his conflict is not inevitable: Dr Carter could arrange his time such that he returned home one or two days earlier, thus mitigating the worst effects of the long-haul flight from Australia. Generally speaking, conflicts of interest that are avoidable require a higher level of justification that those that are unavoidable.

How legitimate are the professional obligations and external interests?

Some interests are more legitimate or justifiable than others. There is never any doubt that professional duties to seek patients' best interests, support high-quality research and education, and promote high standards for the profession are legitimate concerns for doctors to have. In a similar way, certain interests, such as a desire to harm patients or to undermine credible research, are always illegitimate. However, many external interests, while not in and of themselves illegitimate, can become unjustifiable under certain circumstances. In our example above, no one would question that Dr Carter has a legitimate interest in his own welfare, which he expresses by regular holidays in a location that he finds relaxing and satisfying. Nonetheless, the extent to which he pursues this interest arguably makes it unjustifiable.

In many countries, guidelines on financial and commercial dealings in general practice describe circumstances in which a GP's external interest in financial gain would be difficult to justify (World Medical Association 2004). For example, the UK General Medical Council recommends that GPs with financial interests in a residential or nursing home should not usually provide primary care services to patients in that home, unless this is provided under formal NHS commissioning arrangements. While exceptions may arise, these will be rare, and GPs would be expected to justify their actions (General Medical Council 2006b).

How likely is it that professional judgement will be influenced, or appear to be influenced, by external interests?

The likelihood that a GP's professional judgement will be influenced in a conflict of interest is related to a number of factors (Thompson 1993). First, the size of the inducement may be important. At first glance, it seems obvious that the greater the size of the gift, the more likely it is that the GP will be influenced by it. All other things being equal, the conflict of interest that Dr Chu faces by regularly accepting sponsorship to attend overseas conferences seems more serious than that faced by his colleagues who merely eat breakfasts supplied by the pharmaceutical company. However, social science research suggests that the size of the initial gift or favour may not always be important. Some 'small' gifts–'food, friendship and flattery'–can have powerful influences on doctors' behaviour (Blumenthal 2004).

Second, the scope of the conflict is also relevant to the likelihood of influence, in particular as it relates to the nature of the relationship that has created the conflict. For example, a long-standing and close relationship, in which a GP benefits many times from, say, continued support by a pharmaceutical company, is more troubling than one-off gifts. The reasons for this are obvious. Over time, continuing relationships come to generate their own momentum; the GP may enjoy his contact with particular pharmaceutical company representatives and value the relationships he forms. In addition, he may come to depend on the regular gifts, money or support offered by the company. Dr Chu is at risk of being in this situation. Links-Howard regularly sponsors his breakfast meetings and Dr Chu may doubt that he would be able to sustain this activity without the support of the company.

The amount of independence the GP is able to exercise with respect to the judgments he makes is also relevant in a conflict of interest. For example, if there are practice standards that restrict the drugs a GP can prescribe, then that GP is less open to influence by contact with pharmaceutical representatives than one who has total discretion about prescribing practices.

Whatever the factors that influence judgment, it is important for GPs to remember that we are rarely good judges of situations when we stand to benefit ourselves. The social science research literature suggests that human beings have an 'unconscious and unintentional self-serving bias' when it comes to our decisions: we have difficulty recognizing bias in our decisions when that bias will be to our advantage (Dana and Loewenstein 2003).

How serious is the impact of the conflict on the professional obligation?

In evaluating a conflict of interest, it is important to review how seriously any professional duty will be affected. There is often a spectrum of seriousness, ranging from no likelihood of influence (or even a benefit) through to quite serious consequences. For example, consider the possibility that Dr Chu changes his medication regime for specific patients based on his most recent attendance at a conference sponsored by Links-Howard. The change may improve the quality of life of his patients at no greater cost. Alternatively, there may be no improvement or perhaps an increase in annoying side-effects. The new drug may also be more expensive, resulting in increased out-of-pocket expenses for his patients.

Beyond direct impacts on the care of individual patients, Dr Chu needs to think about the more generalized effects of secondary interests. There may be increased costs for the health system overall if he prescribes more costly drugs. Dr Chu may also want to consider the impact that it might have on his patients more generally, should it become known that he is supported by Links-Howard.

Dealing with conflicts of interest

This last point leads naturally to a consideration of remedies for conflict of interest. The remedy most often proposed for conflicts of interest is disclosure to all people who might be affected by the conflict. Alpert has suggested the implementation of a Web-based public registry to address concerns about the relationship between doctors and drug companies. Such a registry would allow everyone, including patients, access to information about the 'level of financial gain and potential conflict of interest' that each doctor has through his or her dealings with pharmaceutical companies (Alpert 2005). This would give people who are likely to be affected by the GP's conflict of interest an opportunity to draw their own conclusions about the likely impact on their wellbeing. Dr Chu could adapt this and begin to deal with his conflict of interest by including in his practice information leaflet a note stating that the practice receives support from the pharmaceutical company, Howard-Links. He could briefly describe the forms that this sponsorship takes and indicate that he is prepared to answer questions about the sponsorship.

Merely disclosing a conflict of interest is rarely a remedy in its own right. 'Disclosing a conflict only reveals a problem, without providing any guidance for resolving it' (Thompson 1993). In fact, all disclosure may do, in the short term, is to increase anxiety, which can undermine trust in the medical profession. If Dr Carter tells his patients that he has just stepped off the plane and that his tiredness may impair his judgment, this is unlikely to inspire patient confidence in his decisions or to contribute to a trusting relationship between GP and patient. Patients who are informed that drug company promotions take place in their practice may question whether other factors also shape the decisions and advice they receive.

The dangers inherent in merely disclosing a conflict of interest do not imply that doctors should keep such conflicts secret. Rather, making others aware of the conflict is really just the first step in addressing the conflict appropriately. The next step is to carefully evaluate the conflict and identify its various components. Thoughtful analysis of the avoidability and legitimacy of the conflict, as well as the likelihood of undue influence and the seriousness of the impact, may lead to a number of outcomes. The conflict may be deemed to be avoidable. Dr Carter's conflict of interest, for example, can be resolved if he returns to the UK from his holiday 24 hours earlier. Dr Chu can refuse to accept sponsorship to travel to conferences at Links-Howard's expense. And, Dr Grainger can request that the payment he receives for his participation in the clinical trial reflect more accurately the time and resources he and his patients put into the trial. Alternatively, analysis of the conflict may suggest that the external interest is illegitimate. Some secondary interests can immediately be dismissed as unethical. Interests which may lead to harm and lack of respect for patients, or which may undermine the integrity of research, fall into this category.

Some conflicts of interest are neither avoidable, nor totally unjustifiable. We then need to think about the likelihood of undue influence and the seriousness of the impact. The onus here is on showing that external interests–for example, financial gain, prestige or public recognition–will *not* exert an undue influence on primary obligations to care for patients and support good research, and that the impact such external interests have will be minor.

Occasionally, GPs will encounter situations either of conflict between professional obligations or where external interests are justifiably powerful. Dr Walker's dilemma concerning the availability of antivirals for her family in a pandemic may be such a situation. In these situations, the GP may need to recognize that her loyalties are unavoidably divided and that she cannot get it completely right. O'Neill, writing in a slightly different context, suggests that:

> Where existing realities may force hard choices, it may be impossible to meet all of the various requirements .... The unmeetable requirement may have 'remainders' and remainders are often viewed as calling for expressions of attitudes such as regret or remorse .... More active responses might include expressions of apology, commitment to reform, the provision of compensation, forms of restitution, making good, and the like.
>
> (O'Neill 2001, p.22)

Just because we cannot reconcile conflicts of interest on all occasions does not mean that we should avoid choosing one over the other in individual instances. GPs may need to make a choice, and note that the choice is imperfect.

One solution that is not likely to work in a conflict of interest is keeping the conflict secret. One helpful way to think about this is to apply the 'front page' test: 'Would [you] mind seeing an article on the front page of your [local] newspaper describing this behaviour?' (Alpert 2005). GPs who are tempted to keep conflicts of interest hidden should bear in mind what is likely to happen should patients and other interested parties learn that the conflict has been concealed. If patients learn that their doctor's secondary interests, such as financial gain, have influenced decisions regarding their treatment, and that the doctor has taken steps to keep this information secret, this is far more likely to harm the doctor–patient relationship than early disclosure.

Consider, for example, the situation of Mr Shawlands and his participation in Dr Grainger's clinical trial. Mr Shawlands is likely to feel annoyed when he learns that Dr Grainger has a financial interest in the trial. It makes little difference if Dr Grainger's principal motive for enrolling patients in the trial is to advance the state of scientific knowledge. The appearance of a conflict of interest is enough to generate concern, and the fact that Dr Grainger's financial gain has been kept secret from his patients can only exacerbate Mr Shawlands' loss of faith in Dr Grainger.

It can be difficult for GPs caught up in conflicts of interest to stand back and evaluate their involvement impartially. For this reason, at the very least, any

GP involved in a conflict of interest should seek advice from an experienced and independent colleague. In some cases, contact with the GP's medical defence organization or the state or national Medical Council or Board may be prudent. In addition, there are certain situations in which review and authorization by independent organizations is required. For example, in many countries GPs who take part in research may only accept payments that have been approved by a Research Ethics Committee.

Conclusion

In this chapter we have explored a wide range of ethical problems that can grouped together as examples of conflicts of interest. We have suggested that thinking about these conflicts as clashes between professional obligations and external interests is helpful. We have also indicated that such conflicts can be evaluated by considering the avoidability and legitimacy of the conflict, as well as the likelihood of undue influence and the seriousness of the impact. Disclosure is generally an important first step in beginning to address a conflict of interest, but often it will not be the sole action a GP needs to take.

References

Alpert JS (2005). Doctors and the drug industry: how can we handle potential conflicts of interest? *American Journal of Medicine* **118**, 99–100.

Blumenthal D (2004). Doctors and drug companies. *New England Journal of Medicine* **351**, 1885–1890.

Chren MM and Landefeld S (1994). Physicians' behaviour and their interactions with drug companies. *Journal of the American Medical Association* **271**, 684–689.

Dana J and Loewenstein G (2003). A social science perspective on gifts to physicians from industry. *Journal of the American Medical Association* **290**, 252–255.

Davis M (2001). Introduction. In Davis M (ed.) *Conflict of interest in the professions*, 3–19. New York, Oxford University Press.

General Medical Council (2006a). *Good medical practice*. GMC, London.

General Medical Council (2006b). *Conflicts of interest*. GMC, London. Available at http://www.gmc-uk.org/guidance/current/library/conflicts_of_interest.asp (accessed 28 February 2008).

Goold SD (2000). Conflicts of interest and obligation. In Sugarman J (ed.) *20 common problems–ethics in primary care*. McGraw-Hill, New York, 93–101.

Gosden T, Forland F, Kristiansen IS, Sutton M, Leese B, Giuffrida A, Sergison M, Pedersen L (2001). Impact of payment method on behaviour of primary care physicians: a systematic review. *Journal of Health Services Research and Policy* **6**(1), 44–55.

Kassirer JP and Angell M (1993). Financial conflicts of interest in biomedical research. *New England Journal of Medicine* **329**, 570–571.

Komesaroff PA and Kerridge IH (2002). Ethical issues concerning the relationship between medical practitioners and the pharmaceutical industry. *Medical Journal of Australia* **176**, 118–121.

Lemmens T and Singer PA (1998). Bioethics for clinicians: Conflicts of interest in research, education and patient care. *CMAJ* **159**, 960–965.

O'Neill O (2001). Practical principles and practical judgement. *Hasting Center Report* **3**, 15–23.

Osgood BS, Krasny AJ and Emanuel LL (2000). Consultation and referral. In Sugarman J (ed.) *20 common problems–ethics in primary care*. McGraw-Hill, New York, 103–115.

Palmer N, Braunack-Mayer A, Rogers W, Provis C and Cullity G (2006). Conflicts of interest in Divisions of General Practice. *Journal of Medical Ethics* **32**, 715–717.

Pellegrino ED (1987). Altruism, self-interest, and medical ethics. *JAMA* **258**, 1939–1940.

Pellegrino ED (1994). Self-interest, the physician's duties and medical ethics: a philosophical and theological challenge. In Campbell CS and Lustig BA (ed.) *Duties to others*. Kluwer Academic Publishers, Netherlands, 125–141.

Raniga S, Hider P, Spriggs D and Ardagh M (2005). Attitudes of hospital medical practitioners to the mandatory reporting of professional misconduct. *Journal of the New Zealand Medical Association* **118**, U1781.

Rhodes R, Cohen N (2001). Misconduct and whistleblowing. Abusing alcohol or drugs, in Kushner T. Thomasma D. (eds.) *Ward Ethics. Cases in Bioethics*. Cambridge, Cambridge Univerisity Press, 201–219.

Thompson DF (1993). Understanding financial conflicts of interest. *NEJM* **329**, 573–576.

Tonelli MR (2007). Conflict of interest in clinical practice. *Chest* **132**, 664–670.

Weber J (2001). Commentary–conflicts of interest. In Kushner T K and Thomasma DC (ed.) *Ward ethics. Dilemmas for medical students and doctors in training*. Cambridge University Press, Cambridge, 208–210.

World Health Organization, Department of Ethics, Equity, Trade and Human Rights (2007). *Ethical considerations in developing a public health response to pandemic influenza*. World Health Organization, Geneva.

World Medical Association (2006). *Statement on professional responsibility for standards of medical care*. Available at http: //www.wma.net/e/policy/m8.htm (accessed 14 February 2008).

World Medical Association (2004). *The World Medical Association statement concerning the relationship between physicians and commercial enterprises*. WMA, Tokyo. Available at http: //www.wma.net/e/policy/r2.htm (accessed 28 February 2008).

Chapter 13

On being a good doctor: virtues in general practice

Introduction

What is a good doctor? Whenever and wherever this question is asked, it sparks debate. In 2002, the *British Medical Journal* ran a series of articles on the nature of good doctoring and recent articles in the *Medical Journal of Australia* (Breen 2007; Irvine 2007) and the *New Zealand Medical Journal* (Patterson 2006) have raised similar issues. Patients also are interested in the answer to this question, not least because a number of recent cases around the world have eroded public confidence in doctoring.

Just what is a good doctor? And, more specifically, what is a good general practitioner? This chapter explores this question, drawing on virtue theory, a branch of ethics that is explicitly concerned with human character and ideas about goodness (and badness) in human beings.

What is different about a virtues approach to ethics in general practice?

So far in this book we have given an account of ethics in general practice that has emphasized '*doing* the right thing'; for example, in the realm of doing what's best for the patient or respecting patient autonomy. But some philosophers do not think that all of ethical practice can be explained by focusing just on what we do. The kinds of people we are, the character traits we have, our intentions and motives, are all important for a complete account of what living an ethically good life involves. And some of these concepts are hard to capture within a definition of ethics that concentrates exclusively on what we do.

Here are two simple examples by way of illustration.

Case 13.1

Dr Mackenzie is leaving his surgery late Friday evening. It has been a long day and he is tired, grumpy and he has a headache. If he could wave a magic wand, he would walk out the door of his practice and never comes back. As he is leaving, the phone rings. He hesitates and then picks it up. Mrs Lonsdale is at the other end, worried about her son James. Dr Mackenzie's demeanour is polite, calm and focused. He asks a few questions and decides that he really ought to see James.

Dr Mackenzie's behaviour is exactly what we would expect of a morally excellent doctor, yet his actions here are not taken after a lengthy period of self-reflection during which he is able to weigh up what the best thing to do in this situation might be. Dr Mackenzie responds *intuitively* with patience and fortitude. He does not let his tiredness or frustration show and he treats Mrs Lonsdale exactly as he would have done had she been the first patient he saw after his annual holiday. We probably think that this is how Dr Mackenzie usually behaves (even though we may be at a loss to understand how he achieves this). Somehow or other, he has learnt to respond to situations like this in a morally exemplary manner.

Now, consider a rather different situation.

Case 13.2

Dr Amy Walker joined the St Andrews Surgery in Dunedin 5 years after graduating with honours from medical school. She appears to be an exemplary doctor. Her technical knowledge and skills are superb and she knows how to use them appropriately in a general practice setting. The patients value her greatly: she listens carefully, is respectful and offers advice judiciously. What's more, she is considerate and thoughtful in her dealings with the staff of the practice, while being appropriately assertive. One evening Dr Mackenzie invites Amy and her husband, Hugh, over for a meal. After dinner, talk turns to why people become doctors and how they get to be the sort of doctors they are. Dr Mackenzie rehearses his own reasons for studying medicine, mumbling something about wanting to help people, while doing something scientific. He mentions his belief that people are 'all the same, underneath' and says that he tries to treat patients as equals. 'Although I've got a lot more skills in some areas than a lot of the patients, they've got a lot of skills that I haven't got. I mean, if a man is a plumber I wouldn't know how to begin to clear a drain out, would I?'

> **Case 13.2** *(continued)*
>
> When Dr Mackenzie asks Dr Walker about her reasons for becoming a doctor, he is stunned by the reply: 'I only became a doctor to make money, and that still really determines how I do things. I realized early on that doctors who appear kind, thoughtful and considerate, who try to fit in with their colleagues, who communicate well, do better. If I didn't think it was in my interests, I'd give up being nice to patients tomorrow.'
>
> (Adapted from Veatch 1985, pp.329–345).

There is something deeply disturbing about Dr Walker, a doctor who does all the right things, but for reasons that appear, intuitively, to be wrong.

Both examples illustrate that our attitudes, motives, characters and fundamental dispositions to behave in certain ways are all morally relevant. Virtue theory is concerned with just these issues. It offers a vehicle to incorporate ideas about character and motives into an account of ethics in general practice.

What is virtue ethics?

Virtue ethics is concerned with the kinds of abilities and attitudes we need to have to be able to act morally. The focus, as we noted above, is on character and therefore on the way in which morally good people respond to situations. Virtue theorists hold the view that what makes an action right is that it is done by someone of virtuous character. In one fell swoop this simple observation shifts our attention quite dramatically from the things that a person does to what that person is like–their character, their settled ways of doing things, their personality traits.

In a general practice context, a virtue ethics approach asks: what kind of person is a morally good GP? At an intuitive level, we all can answer this question by listing off character traits that we think are good, worthwhile or virtuous. We may think, generally, of things such as honesty, trustworthiness, benevolence, respectfulness, courage and integrity. Some of these characteristics we have already discussed elsewhere in this book. We dealt with the concept of trust and the trustworthy doctor at length in Chapter 3, and the philosophical and practical aspects of beneficence and respect for autonomy in Chapters 6 and 8. Chapter 7 considered how fairness might be practised in a general practice setting. In the following section of this chapter we want to consider one more virtue, which we think is especially important in a general practice context: the virtue of compassion.

Compassion

GPs frequently encounter suffering in their work and they have many ways to deal with it. Some GPs practise a form of 'detached concern', building a barrier between themselves and their patients that recognizes the pain but refuses to let it touch them (Brody 1998). Less commonly, there are GPs whose experience of their patients' misfortunes almost seems to mimic the patients' suffering. Then there are a small group of doctors whose defence mechanisms are so well-developed that they no longer see suffering at all.

Such responses are not part of the practice of the virtuous doctor. Rather, the virtuous doctor responds to suffering with compassion. We think that compassion is a particularly important virtue for general practice, because it offers GPs a way to manage their ongoing contact with apparently inexplicable instances of illness, suffering, death and misfortune *and* the pull of those instances on their emotions.

Just what is involved in being a compassionate GP? We suggest that compassion has four characteristics (Nussbaum 1996; Blum 1997).

The compassionate GP focuses on people who are suffering

Compassion is a response to pain or suffering in others. The person for whom compassion is felt must be suffering a harm, be in some difficulty or be in danger. The suffering also needs to be reasonably serious or, at least, not trivial. Compassion is typically evoked when we see death, pain or serious illness, all things that are part and parcel of the GP's daily work.

It is important to note here that the GP who feels compassion does not simply accept other people's judgments about the seriousness of their suffering. The compassionate GP has her own point of view on the suffering she sees. She doesn't necessarily agree to see things as her patient sees them; in fact, she may ascribe a rather different value to what she sees happening to a patient. This independence of judgment can cut two ways. First, the GP may not necessarily think her patient's misfortune is as significant as he thinks it is. For example, when otherwise fit and healthy John comes to see his GP complaining loudly of a sore throat of 24 hours duration, we hardly expect the GP's response to be compassion. On the other hand, a compassionate GP can also 'feel for' the patient who seems unaware that his situation warrants compassion. Imagine an elderly man caring, with little support, for his dying wife. The GP can see that the husband's physical and psychological health is suffering; yet, the man refuses to accept help and will not even acknowledge that what he is doing is out of the ordinary. Rather, he sees this as 'just doing what has to be done'. He may not think his situation makes him worthy of compassion; we would probably agree with the GP that it does.

Compassion involves imagining what the suffering must be like

Compassion is obviously much more than just an attitude directed toward a person who is suffering, because indifference or curiosity are also attitudes that can be directed at people who suffer. We do occasionally meet health professionals who seem to adopt this disengaged, but interested, attitude towards patients who are clearly in psychological or physical pain. We may wonder whether there is something 'missing' in their attitude or approach to patients; that something is compassion.

Being compassionate means that we actively try to imagine what it must be like to be suffering as this patient is suffering. This is not the same as 'identifying' with the patient, where the emphasis is rather more on what I would feel if I were in that situation. Identifying involves blurring the boundaries between the GP and the patient, such that the GP can no longer really tell where the patient's experience ends and the GP's begins. Nor does the capacity to imagine the other's condition require that a GP have experienced in the past what his patient is experiencing now, although prior experience may certainly help us to imagine what it is like for other people.

Martha Nussbaum frames this imaginative reconstruction in a rather different way and calls it 'a judgment of *similar possibilities*' (Nussbaum 1996, p.34). She emphasizes that this does not mean that a compassionate GP should suffer *with* patients. Rather, the GP always sees herself as separate from the patient, while recognizing that the pain, illness, misfortune that the patient is experiencing could, under different conditions, happen to her.

The fact that compassion judges another's suffering to be possible for oneself is what sets it apart from the response of intellectual curiosity or indifference. The compassionate onlooker knows that goods such as food, health, freedom, etc., *do* matter, and that none of us are immune from having these goods taken away from us. Compassion is one of those virtues that help us to cross class, nationality, race and gender boundaries; the compassionate person 'assumes these different positions in imagination, and comes to see the obstacles to flourishing faced by human beings in these many concrete situations' (Nussbaum 1996, p.51).

Being able to accept other people's suffering as possibilities for ourselves is what allows compassion to be a 'bridge between the individual and the community' (Nussbaum 1996, p.28). That bridge involves regarding the other people as human beings, like us, and it means acknowledging that there is some sense in which we are equal. It is exemplified in the way Dr Mackenzie, at the beginning of this chapter, attempted to define his relationship with his patients: 'we're all the same, underneath'. It may help to see why this sense of shared humanity is important to compassion if we think about situations in which it is absent. It is hard to imagine feeling compassion for someone whom we regard as superior to, or above, ourselves in some way, and it is pity, rather than compassion, that we feel for someone whom we think is inferior or below us in some way. In both cases, we deem the other person 'fundamentally different' from ourselves.

Because compassion has this quality of imaginative reconstruction of others' experiences, people who find it hard to imagine other ways of seeing, doing and being things tend to be less compassionate. It is also why some doctors will say that, as they become older, they feel the pull of compassion more deeply. This may be, at least in part, because their broader life experiences create a greater awareness of what life is like for other people.

Compassion involves active concern for the wellbeing of others

Compassion makes no sense unless it is tied to caring about and, usually, trying to alleviate the suffering that we observe. The compassionate doctor does much more than acknowledge and interpret her patients' suffering. She also cares that they are suffering and she wants to do something about that suffering. Often, there will be much that she can do. She can attempt to find the cause of the pain, discomfort and suffering; she can offer treatment and advice for self-management. Here, the motive for her actions will not be primarily that it makes her feel better (although that may well be the case), but that it will improve things for her patients.

Compassion is a driver for beneficent actions towards patients. We can see very clearly here the difference between the action of doing good and the intentions and motives that drive those actions. Amy Walker behaves beneficently–she acts for the good of her patients–but she lacks compassion, for her motives ultimately concern only herself.

Ironically, compassion has a particularly important role to play when we cannot manage to alleviate suffering. The compassionate person is optimistic: she continues to hope that something will work to lessen the suffering or to allay the fears. Merely being with people in their suffering can make a difference, and many patients will testify to how much it did help to have their GP just 'being with them'. Moreover, because a compassionate doctor continues to care in the face of apparent defeat, she is more open to unexpected or unlikely sources of relief for patients. Compassion carries with it a sense of never giving up. This does not mean refusing to recognize terminal illness or endlessly striving for a cure, but rather never giving up on the patient.

Compassion is an enduring emotion

Compassion is not a transient attitude which is here today, gone tomorrow. Like other virtues, it is characterized by its enduring quality; it is a trait that we develop and exhibit over a long period of time. Again, it is easy to see why this is the case if one considers expressions of concern that are more fleeting. The momentary twinges of conscience some of us feel when we contemplate the victims of an earthquake or a famine on the other side of the world may indicate our concern for the plight of others. However, unless those twinges develop into something more lasting, we would hardly describe our response as compassion.

Limits to compassion

Compassion, when understood wrongly or practised inappropriately, can actually cause harm. Patients may be harmed by a GP who is over-compassionate, as this may encourage the patient to focus too much on his illness. GPs may be harmed if compassion leads to an exclusive focus on one patient's suffering to the detriment of other patients, or if it blinds the GP to a more balanced way of seeing things. Like all of the virtues, compassion is not a virtue to be practised in isolation. In particular, compassion must be tempered with the following:

- respectfulness–to maintain a sense of patients as independent and able to chart their own course;
- justice–to ensure that all patients are treated fairly, with due consideration given to each person who needs it; and
- beneficence–to keep what is in the patient's best interests in the forefront at all times and, in particular, to ensure that knowledge and reason prevail.

Medical vices

If there can be virtues in and for general practice, there can also be vices. A number of other writers also refer to vices in medicine, generally by way of contrast with the virtues (Drane 1994). One way to frame a discussion of the vices, is in terms of commitments. Medical vices are character traits that accompany the wrong kinds of ultimate commitments: to money, to power, to scienc, or to self. We will look at each of these briefly.

There is a long, and sometimes unpleasant, history behind descriptions of doctors as 'only in it for the money', but the topic is canvassed only rarely in medical ethics textbooks. Amy Walker, at the beginning of this chapter, is unusual in her forthright commitment to money. To understand what disturbs us about Amy's position, we need to go back to our definition of a virtue. For the problem with being ultimately committed to money is that it cannot lead to lives that are well-lived, either in a general sense or in the more specific form of healing or care for patients. The doctor committed ultimately to money ceases to care for patients when there is no economic benefit for herself. In a similar way, an ultimate commitment to power runs counter to empowering patients or even to working productively in a team with other health professionals.

An ultimate commitment to science might seem a somewhat strange inclusion in a list of vices. What could be wrong with being committed to a medicine that is practised scientifically? The problem is, again, the notion of an ultimate commitment. The GP who is ultimately committed to science risks losing interest in patients when science alone can provide no biological remedies. This is a perilous route for general practice, for, as we have discussed previously, there is much of general practice care that does not turn on scientific evidence and proven treatments. Nor can GPs expect even to be able to offer an effective remedy for all the problems they meet.

Finally, there is the question of having an ultimate commitment to self. We have explored the role of self-interest in our chapter on conflicts of interest. There we suggested that GPs who pursue secondary interests, such as personal gain, power or prestige, risk damaging the relationship of trust that ought to exist between them and their patients. At the end of the moral day, it is Amy Walker's selfishness, her ultimate commitment to self, that most disturbs us. Someone who is turned in on herself cannot really be trusted to pursue the best interests of patients in her care.

Why do we need a focus on virtue in medicine?

We have suggested that compassion is an important virtue for general practice. Along with other virtues, it implies a different way to think about moral goods in general practice. Before we conclude our discussion of virtue, we want to make a few points about the special value of a virtue ethics approach (Pellegrino 1995).

Some writers, such as Edmund Pellegrino, think that we need an emphasis on virtue as a corrective to some current morally questionable practices in medicine–refusing to treat patients with AIDS, turning away the poor, complying with early discharge rules when it is medically inappropriate, medical entrepreneurialism. Perhaps if we concentrated more on selecting, training and encouraging doctors to be virtuous, we would have less of these practices.

Others argue that we need to emphasize virtue because of the specialization and bureaucratization of medicine (May 1994). These factors have meant that we now see very little of what an individual practitioner does, where once the doctor's work was more open to scrutiny. The argument here is clearest if we contrast, say, the practice of a specialist vascular surgeon working in a large city today and that of a general practitioner based in a small rural village fifty years ago. Fifty years ago, an efficient grapevine would have ensured that the country doctor's successes and failures were more widely known than the vascular surgeon's could ever be today. In addition, the country doctor would be the sole recipient of any blame or praise, which is now dispersed widely in institutions, rather than attributed to individuals. A focus on virtue can help protect us against the self-interested physician, who, in a smaller world, would have been scrutinized carefully by a watchful community.

Third, focusing on virtues such as compassion reminds us that good general practice involves far more than technical skill. A virtuous doctor is certainly technically competent: she displays the skills of an applied scientist in combining her clinical expertise with familiarity and appropriate application of the best available evidence. But a virtuous doctor is also more than a sophisticated diagnostic therapeutic machine. A virtuous doctor is humane: he displays the personal qualities that human beings need to assist people in their suffering.

Finally, a virtue ethics approach also encourages us to think about how we become the sort of people we are. Although virtues are, in some ways, intuitive, they are not things 'we find ourselves with, but something we construct over a lifetime' (Drane 1994). Virtues are acquired human qualities, learnt and practised in what we do and how we think about our actions. This component to our description of a virtue suggests that we can learn to be certain kinds of people; we can try to develop certain ways of responding to things and to limit other ways. When an experienced GP says 'one of the things I've had to learn over the years is to control my impatience when people don't catch on as quickly as I do', we see virtue as a practised skill in action.

This notion of the virtues as acquired human qualities also opens up a discussion about the close two-way relationship between character development and the social and cultural environment. The way in which character is formed is obviously influenced by the social settings in which people live. So, how we educate doctors is important, not only for the technical knowledge and skills that are learnt, but also for the values that students acquire during their training. It is well-recognized that there is a hidden curriculum in medical education that impacts powerfully on students' ethical awareness. For example, medical students who learn how to be doctors in impersonal hospital bureaucracies sometimes take from those bureaucracies values that emphasize curing the disease at the price of alleviating the patient's suffering. Andre notes that students' developing 'ability to see the moral landscape' is constrained by a number of factors. She cites the stress and suffering and the 'sometimes desperate lack of time' during medical training as obstacles to clear moral vision (Andre 1992). Students who are occupied for most of the day in lectures, tutorials and ward rounds, and who are overwhelmed and exhausted by the volume of material to be learnt, are too tired, both physically and emotionally, to reflect on what it is that might make a good doctor.

Just as our characters are shaped by the social and cultural environment around us, so we are able to shape that environment ourselves. Our characters can and do contribute to social values and to the moral life of institutions. This is obvious when we meet individuals whose honesty and integrity have exercised a significant influence on the ethos of their work place. For example, many doctors will describe eloquently how, as medical students or junior doctors, their beliefs and values were shaped by their contact with consultants who, through example, exemplified for them what being a good doctor was all about. We might hope that, in a similar way, Dr Mackenzie's belief in the essential equality of human beings and his commitment to helping people might rub off on Amy Walker.

Conclusion: what is a good GP?

We began this chapter with the question 'What is a good general practitioner?'. Throughout this book, we have tried to address this question in various ways. We have suggested that the good GP is trustworthy, discrete, beneficent, respectful, honest, fair and compassionate. A critic might respond to this list by saying that these virtues ought to be upheld by *all* doctors. Are there virtues that are peculiar to general practice? Our answer to this question is that general practice does not have an exclusive claim to particular virtues. However, there are some virtues that seem particularly appropriate in a general practice context. In this concluding section, we return to the definition of general practice we offered in Chapter 1 and use it to sketch out some virtues for general practice.

General practice is distinguished by the central place it gives to the doctor–patient relationship. A number of things flow from this relationship– commitment to the patient as a whole human being, continuity of care over time, comprehensive care and awareness of the patient's place in his or her family and wider community. These characteristics of relationship in general practice in turn suggest particular virtues.

Commitment to the patient as a person involves knowing and understanding the medical, personal, social and psychological circumstances of one's patients.

Jackie Silvers, in Chapter 1, was a beneficiary of her GP's commitment to her as a person.

Case 13.3

Ms Jackie Silvers is a 35-year-old mother of three young children. She lives with her husband, who is an executive with a computer company and who spends a lot of time away from home. Their youngest child has severe asthma and the middle child has extremely aggressive behaviour that has responded only poorly to a series of appointments with a psychologist. Ms Silvers presents on this occasion with recurrent headaches. Dr Buchan knows that her husband is away in the USA on a 3-week trip, and that the youngest child was admitted last week as an emergency with his asthma. Ms Silvers has recently had a promotion in her work and is now managing a team of staff in the local council offices.

Dr Buchan takes a history and examines Ms Silvers. His provisional diagnosis is that these are tension headaches, exacerbated by recent stresses in Ms Silvers' life.

Dr Buchan's knowledge of Ms Silvers as a person helps him to reach a diagnosis and to spare Ms Silvers the inconvenience and anxiety of further investigations. His contact with Ms Silvers involves both action and promise (May 1994). Dr Buchan's actions involve taking a thorough history and conducting a careful examination. His promises may be various, depending on what he feels is appropriate therapeutically and what Ms Silvers wishes– 'There are a number of things we can do to help you', 'I can assure you that this is nothing serious'. Such promises are worthless if Dr Buchan does not follow them through. Therefore, the virtue that Dr Buchan needs to practise here is fidelity, the virtue of being true to one's promises, which is an important part of being trustworthy. And being true to one's promises acquires special poignancy in general practice, because relationships can often last a long time.

The length of relationship between doctor and patient is associated with a second characteristic of general practice–the provision of continuous care. Because GPs provide continuity of care over time they need the virtue of perseverance. Perseverance has at least two facets: it involves the capacity to pursue diligently the concerns that the patient brings, and it requires persistence to stick with a patient when things do not seem to go right. The specialist may return a patient to a GP with the words 'I can't find anything wrong here', but the GP does not have this luxury. His role as the point of continuing contact means that he cannot wash his hands of his patients. May suggests that such behaviour is one of the 'inconspicuous marks of courage' (May 1994, p.86), for perseverance requires that we continue in the face of adversity. In Dr Buchan's case, adversity may show its face in the fact that he is unable to do more than offer band aid solutions to Ms Silvers' problems. Ms Silvers may be a difficult and demanding patient, who implies that Dr Buchan ought to be able to do more for her. It requires considerable courage to continue to care for such a patient.

The third characteristic of relationships in general practice is the comprehensiveness of the care required. GPs must be able to see anything that walks in the door. There are many virtues associated with good comprehensive care—conscientiousness, perseverance and prudence all spring to mind. One virtue that is often forgotten here is the virtue of humility. The lengthy training and specialized knowledge that accompanies being a doctor often brings with it a sense of superiority and patients may pander to this in many ways. Yet, virtuous practice acknowledges, as Dr Mackenzie does at the beginning of this chapter, that there is nothing inherently 'special' about the knowledge and skills of the doctor. The virtuous GP recognizes that people are 'all the same, underneath' and this underpins the attitude of respectfulness that the good GP brings to her work.

Finally, general practice locates patients in the context of their whole lives and acknowledges that patients are, first and foremost, people with hopes, fears and ongoing lives. GPs, more than any other specialty in medicine, have the opportunity to practise the virtues of ordinary, everyday life—trustworthiness, thoughtfulness, patience, generosity, integrity. The list here is endless, but the point of the list is important. At the end of the day, the good GP is a good human being, practising the virtues in a particular setting with the special responsibilities and joys that this brings.

References

Andre J (1992). Learning to see: moral growth during medical training. *Journal of Medical Ethics* **18**, 148–152.

Blum L (1997). Compassion. In Kruschwitz RC and Roberts RB (ed.) *The virtues. Contemporary essays on moral character.* Belmont, California, Wadsworth Publishing Company, 229–238.

Breen KJ (2007). Medical professionalism: is it really under threat? *Medical Journal of Australia* **186**, 596–598.

Brody H (1998). The family physician: what sort of person? *Family Medicine* **30**(8), 589–593.

Drane JF (1994). Character and the moral life. A virtue approach to biomedical ethics. In DuBose ER, Hamel R and O'Connell LJ (ed.). *A matter of principles? Ferment in US bioethics.* Valley Forge, Trinity Press International, 284–309.

Irvine DH (2007). Everyone is entitled to a good doctor. *Medical Journal of Australia* **186**, 256–261.

May W (1994). The virtues in a professional setting. In Fulford KWM, Gillett GR and Soskice JM (ed.) *Medicine and moral reasoning.* New York, Cambridge University Press, 75–90.

Nussbaum M (1996). Compassion: the basic social emotion. *Social Philosophy and Policy* **13**, 27–58.

Paterson R (2006). Leadership in medicine. *The New Zealand Medical Journal* 04 August 2006 119(1239) URL: http://www.nzma.org.nz/journal/119–1239/2098/ (accessed 25 August 2008).

Pellegrino ED (1995). Toward a virtue-based normative ethics for the health professions. *Kennedy Institute of Ethics Journal* **5**, 253–260.

Veatch RM (1985). Against virtue–a deontological critique of virtue theory in medical ethics. In Shelp EE (ed.) *Virtue and medicine.* D Reidel Publishing Company, 329–345.

Index